G000067522

Alan E. Oestreich

Growth of the Pediatric Skeleton
A Primer for Radiologists

Alan E. Oestreich

Growth of the Pediatric Skeleton

A Primer for Radiologists

With illustrations by

Tamar Kahane Oestreich

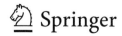 Springer

ALAN E. OESTREICH, MD, FACR
Radiology 5031
Cincinnati Children's Hospital Medical Center
3333 Burnett Ave.
Cincinnati OH 45229-3039
USA

Library of Congress Control Number: 2007933312

ISBN 978-3-540-37688-0 Springer Berlin Heidelberg New York

This work is subject to copyright. All rights are reserved, whether the whole or part of the material is concerned, specifically the rights of translation, reprinting, reuse of illustrations, recitations, broadcasting, reproduction on microfilm or in any other way, and storage in data banks. Duplication of this publication or parts thereof is permitted only under the provisions of the German Copyright Law of September 9, 1965, in its current version, and permission for use must always be obtained from Springer-Verlag. Violations are liable for prosecution under the German Copyright Law.

Springer is part of Springer Science+Business Media

http//www.springer.com
© Springer-Verlag Berlin Heidelberg 2008
Printed in Germany

The use of general descriptive names, trademarks, etc. in this publication does not imply, even in the absence of a specific statement, that such names are exempt from the relevant protective laws and regulations and therefore free for general use.

Product liability: The publishers cannot guarantee the accuracy of any information about dosage and application contained in this book. In every case the user must check such information by consulting the relevant literature.

Medical Editor: Dr. Ute Heilmann, Heidelberg
Desk Editor: Wilma McHugh, Heidelberg
Production Editor: Kurt Teichmann, Mauer
Cover-Design: Frido Steinen-Broo, eStudio Calmar, Spain
Typesetting: Verlagsservice Teichmann, Mauer

Printed on acid-free paper – 21/3180xq – 5 4 3 2 1 0

Dedicated to the memory of
our parents

Edith and Mitchell Oestreich
Elfriede and Peter Kahane

Introduction

Welcome. After years of studying radiographs of the growing bones in children, I would like to put down in print some of the things I have learned about principles of bone growth. I would also like to relate how these principles can help explain some of the abnormalities that are seen in disease and in abnormalities of bone growth. In this effort I am fortunate to be able to draw upon the illustrative abilities of Tamar Kahane Oestreich, my dear wife. Because she insists on understanding what I am trying to have appear on the page, her drawings should help you understand as well (Fig. 1: basic drawing).

Principles and results that can be adduced from the appearance of bones on plain radiographs are emphasized, together with information known from the histology of bone. The tons of information that lurk behind the things we see on radiographs of growing bones in terms of biochemistry, genetics, and related disciplines are not the subject of this little book. Nevertheless, you and I should be aware of their existence and the importance of the scientific progress that is being made in these fields. Occasionally, I will mention at least hox genes or even apoptosis.

Growth makes bones larger and it also makes them change in appearance as they develop. Normal and abnormal bones arise either from the cartilaginous growth plate, a pretty fancy item, or from membrane, which is a more straightforward system.

We thank Dr. Ute Heilmann of Springer-Verlag, for her encouragement, as well as Dr. Heilmann, Annette Hinze and Wilma McHugh of Springer-Verlag, for their assistance in the editorial process.

Some of our major ideas about bone growth in children appeared in a series of articles in the journal, *Skeletal Radiology*:

Oestreich AE, Ahmad BS (1992) The Periphysis and Its Effect on the Metaphysis: I. Definition and Normal Radiographic Pattern. Skeletal Radiol 21:283–286

Oestreich AE, Ahmad BS (1993) The Periphysis and Its Effect on the Metaphysis: II. Application to Rickets and Other Abnormalities. Skeletal Radiol 22:115–120

Oestreich AE, The Acrophysis (2003) A Unifying Concept for Understanding Enchondral Bone Growth and Its Disorders. I. Normal Growth. Skeletal Radiol 32:121–127

Oestreich AE: The Acrophysis (2004) A Unifying Concept for Understanding Enchondral Bone Growth and Its Disorders: II. Abnormal Growth. Skeletal Radiol 33:119–128

Our journey through bone growth now gets underway. Please learn and enjoy as well.

Fig. 1. Artist rendition of three basic bone types in childhood. The longest, based on the left femur, represents a tubular bone with epiphyses at both ends; the intermediate sized bone, based on a 2nd metacarpal, represents a tubular bone with an epiphysis at only one end; and the smallest, based on a capitate, represents a bone growing exclusively by enchondral growth. For a bone with only membranous growth, see Figure 60, the vomer.

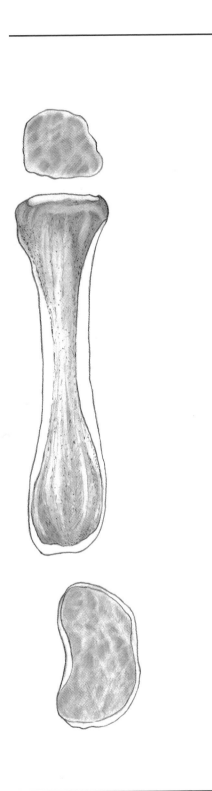
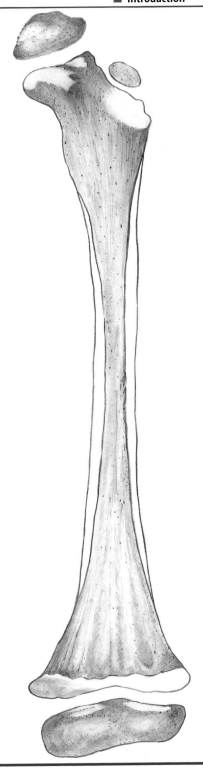

Contents

1

The Two Types of Bone Formation

Bone grows in two ways in humans (and mammals, as well as other related animals). In *enchondral bone growth*, bone arises from columns of cartilage cells in growth plates which undergo a well-defined sequence of activities and changes in morphology. This results in a zone of provisional calcification which, by means of vascular invasion, then becomes bone. In *membranous bone growth*, bone does not arise from cartilage but rather from membrane, fibrous tissue, or mesenchyme.

The duality of bone formation, *enchondral* vs. *membranous*, underlines a large number of differences during normal and abnormal growth. Some bones are purely one or the other in origin. However, many bones arise from both enchrondral and membranous growth, and for these latter bones the interrelations of each system also need to be understood (Fig. 2).

The shape of bones, most notably tubular bones, is influenced by the relative rates of enchondral and membranous growth. Especially the contours at metaphyses and diametaphyses are a consequence of the relative speeding or slowing of enchondral growth compared to membranous growth (Fig. 3). Thus, when enchondral growth alone is slowed, the bones appear to be thicker, while actually they are shorter with normal width. More locally, the concavity of the margins of the diametaphyses (on a frontal radiograph, the medial and lateral margins) depends on those rates (Fig. 4). In achondroplasia, for example, the concavity is greater (i.e., shorter radius of curvature) than normal; in part, because the longitudinal distance between physis and shaft is shorter.

The terminology of that concavity as it appears in the literature (i.e., over-tubulation and undertubulation) is highly inconsistent and confusing. Some

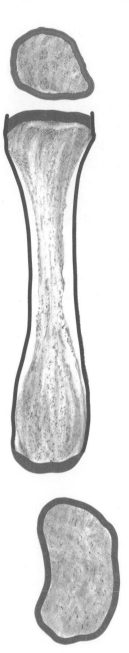

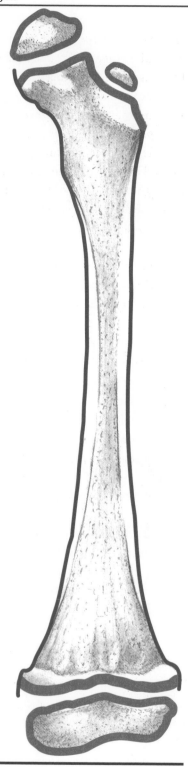

Fig. 2. Sites of enchondral (*red*) and membranous (*blue*) bone growth for the three basic bones from Fig. 1. Red indicates enchondral zones of provisional calcification from physes and their equivalents (acrophyses); blue indicates membranous periosteal-origin bone and bone bark.

persons refer to the greater concavity of achondroplasia as being overtubulation while others call it undertubulation. Consequently, I would recommend avoiding the terms altogether.

In the tubular bones at the physis and metaphysis, the coupling of enchondral and membranous growth is shaped by the metaphyseal collar, which I call **periphysis**. This is a layer, one cell in thickness, called **bone bark**. It encircles the more mature portions of the growth plate (toward the diaphysis) and the few millimeters of most recent growth of the metaphysis (Fig. 5). Through the course of time, the collar allows transverse widening of this region and simultaneously limits that widening so that growth proceeds no swifter than at a determined pace. In the case of the dysplasia metatropic dysplasia, however, the collar seems to abdicate its restraint on transverse growth. A result of the periphysis collar is that the contour of the most recently formed metaphysis is longitudinally straight for a few millimeters (usually 1–3 mm for the long bones) before the bone begins its monotonically curved outer contour. Enchondral growth plates other than the physes themselves do not have a similar membranous collar. More detail on the periphysis may be found in my references listed in the Introduction of this book.

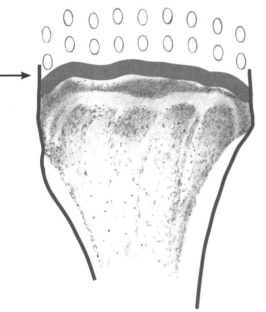

Fig. 3. Diagram of the metaphyseal region. The membranous, one-cell-thick, bone bark (arrow) lies peripheral to the physeal columns of cartilage cells near the metaphysis, as well as peripheral to the cartilaginous zone of provisional calcification (*red*) and the primary spongiosa beyond it.

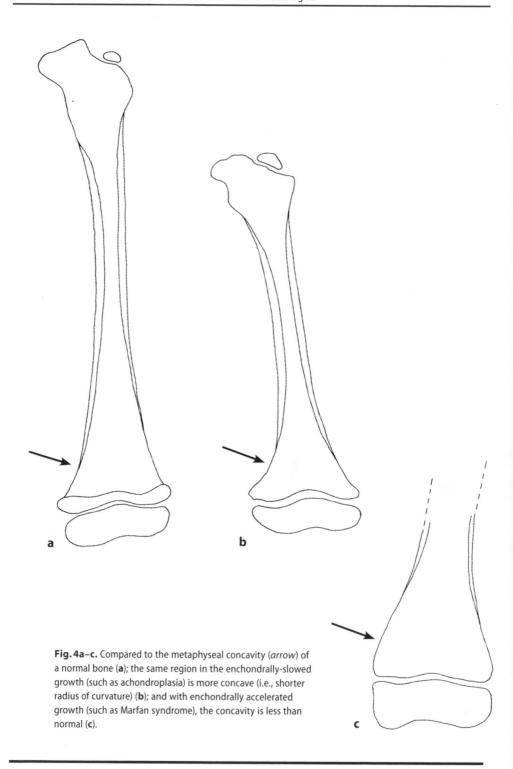

Fig. 4a–c. Compared to the metaphyseal concavity (*arrow*) of a normal bone (**a**); the same region in the enchondrally-slowed growth (such as achondroplasia) is more concave (i.e., shorter radius of curvature) (**b**); and with enchondrally accelerated growth (such as Marfan syndrome), the concavity is less than normal (**c**).

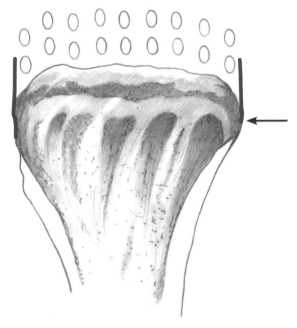

Fig. 5. The one-cell-thick bone bark (*blue*) gives a distinctive shape to the periphysis region, ending in a step-off (*arrow*) between straight metaphysis and the curve of the shaft.

2

Enchondral Growth: Physes and Acrophyses

Enchondral growth occurs not only at the physis growth plates but also at many other sites of enchondral growth.

I have coined the term *"acrophysis"* to describe the normal growth plates situated at all sites of the skeleton other than the classic physes. This term serves to emphasize the similarities and differences of enchondral growth at the varied sites (Fig. 6). Epiphyses and their equivalents, including carpals, tarsals, sesamoids, and apophyses, all develop solely by enchondral growth and are thus surrounded by acrophyses, each of which interfaces with the already ossified center/bone at its zone of provisional calcification. The non-epiphyseal end of proximal and middle phalanges also have an acrophysis. (It is thought that the terminal tufts of distal phalanges may also arise from an acrophysis but this has not yet been verified).

Do epiphyses or carpals have a cortex? If cortex is meant to signify a limiting rim of **bone**, such as along the shafts of tubular bones (Fig. 7), then epiphyses, carpals, tarsals, and sesamoids do not have a cortex (at least not in childhood), since their limiting radiodense rim is the zone of provisional calcification **cartilage**. By this definition, the apposing edges of cranial flat bones, although formed in membrane, do not qualify as cortex.

The *pseudoepiphysis*, most frequently seen at the proximal end of the second metacarpal, is separated from the main shaft by a soft tissue density cleft that behaves as fibrous tissue rather than enchondral cartilage (Fig. 8). Its incidence depends on how minor a cleft is included within your definition. Non-minimal pseudoepiphyses are seen in second metacarpals in Southern Ohio in up to 25% of normal children; less frequently in London, UK, and from the films we have observed, even less frequently in Tibet. A higher frequency of pseudoepiphyses of second metacarpals and other tubular bones is seen in some dysostoses and syndromes, most prominently in cleido-cranial dysplasia.

Enchondral growth at physes and acrophyses is programmed so that the rate of growth depends on the site. For example, the most rapid physis is at the distal femur. Changes in rates of growth, such as slowing in achondroplasia, affects most prominently the sites of normal greatest growth, so that the largest bones are the most shortened ones, compared to normal children. Each long bone has a relative rate of growth different at its proximal and its distal end. The rates are reflected in the position of growth arrest/recovery lines or lead lines, compared to the physis. The faster the growth, the further they lie from the physis (Fig. 9). Radius growth, for example, is greater at the distal end than the proximal end. The same markers indicate the relative rates of acrophyseal growth in growth centers and their equivalents, such as tarsal bones. When increased local vascularity speeds maturation, the separation of these lines from the physis will increase; when growth is tethered or vascularity decreases, the separation decreases, and indeed, the absence of growth at a site means no growth recovery can occur at that site.

Cysts of long bone shafts seem to "grow" away from the physis once they are no longer in continuity with it. Of course, what is actually happening is that normal enchondral bone is progressively developing between the cyst and the physis.

However, enchondromas generally remain in contact with the physis from which they "arise"; no ossification of the former physeal cartilage has occurred. Consequently, a tube of cartilage grows and remains as cartilage, while the bone next to the tube does grow.

Prior to any ossification, enchondral sites have a cartilaginous presence which can be detected, for example, by ultrasound or MRI. Purely membranous bones have a mesenchymal model prior to the onset of ossification.

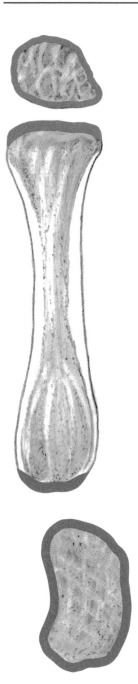
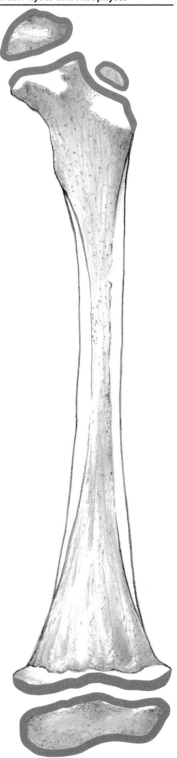

Fig. 6. Red indicates the enchondral cartilaginous zones of provisional calcification, not only from physeal cartilage, but also from acrophyseal enchondral sites (width of the zones not to scale).

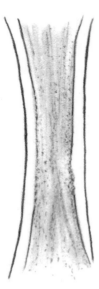

Fig. 7. Cortex of tubular bone, shown in white, is formed at periosteal membranous bone sites.

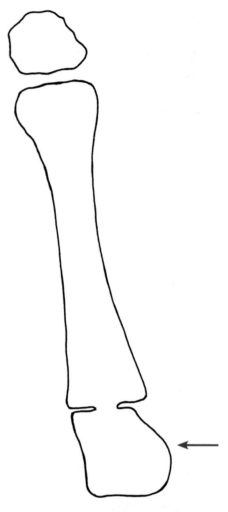

Fig. 8. Pseudoepiphysis (*arrow*), shown here as moderately prominent, forms at the non-epiphyseal end of short tubular bones, especially the 2nd metacarpal. When it is even more complete, it gives that end of the bone an appearance similar to a true epiphysis.

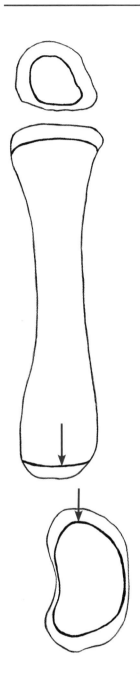

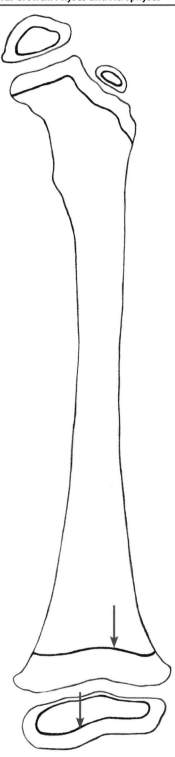

Fig. 9. Growth arrest/recovery lines form beyond each site of enchondral growth (several are indicated here by arrows). The distance from the physis or acrophysis depends on the rate of enchondral growth at that site.

3 Membranous Growth

Many of the bones of the skull and face are all membranous in origin. Tubular bones and certain "deformed tubular bones," such as scapula and bones of the bony pelvis, are partly membranous and partly enchondral in origin, as are some of the bones of the skull base.

The two sites of membranous bone growth of tubular bones differ somewhat in nature, although both consist of bone arising from membrane without the intervention of enchondral growth. Better known is bone arising along the shaft, which, as is the case with membranous flat bones, arises from periosteum (Fig. 10). The other site is at the metaphysis and physis of tubular bones, where a metaphyseal collar is present in which a layer of bone, one cell in thickness, arises that allows transverse growth, and yet at the same time also restricts transverse growth from happening too rapidly (Fig. 10). This one-cell-thick layer is known as bone bark and lies peripheral to the distal portions of the physis as well as the straight area (usually 1–3 mm long) of the metaphysis, the most recently formed metaphysis.

The shafts of tubular bones, especially long bones, respond to heavy muscular activity with a thicker cortex and wider bone, whereas, muscular weakness or inactivity leads to slender bones with thin cortex and often osteoporotic bone. In general, increased vascularity means increased bone growth in childhood. Presumably, such increased vascularity plays a role in dysplasias and dysostoses with thick cortices, such as progressive diaphyseal dysplasia, i.e., Engelmann disease.

The portion of fracture healing that occurs under the periosteum is mebranous bone formation. Generally, the ossification proceeds from the peri-

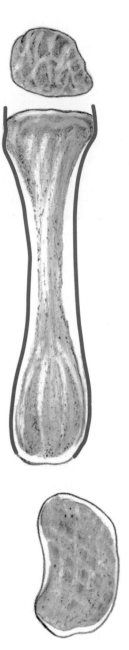
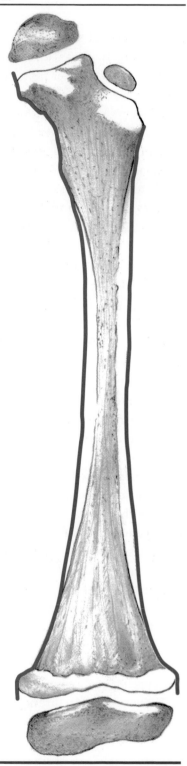

Fig. 10. The sites of membranous bone growth are indicated in blue, arising from periosteum along shafts and as bone bark at the periphysis. Note that growth centers and carpal (and tarsal) bones have no membranous growth (and no periosteum).

osteum most distant from the actual fracture site and then inward toward the fracture. Healing within a bone is by endosteal callus not from the periosteum. Bones without periosteum do not get periosteal reaction. So don't believe someone who says the lunate shows periosteal reaction.

In the surgical technique of ***corticotomy***, an incision is made through periosteum. The cut, however, is mainly made through bone cortex (hence "corticotomy"), sparing the periosteum as much as possible. Therefore, membranous bone growth remains available to make bone in the gap that is created when the bone is stretched. Similarly, during scoliosis surgery, portions of ribs may be removed while leaving the periosteum so that the ribs will regenerate. These are practical uses of understanding membranous bone formation.

In several ways the line of dense bone surrounding unerupted teeth and around the roots of erupted teeth, the ***lamina dura*** (Fig. 11), resembles cortex of tubular bones. For example, it becomes washed out and even invisible in established hyperparathyroidism. Just as cortex is breached as osteomyelitis escapes from the marrow cavity of bone, periapical abscess from tooth infec-

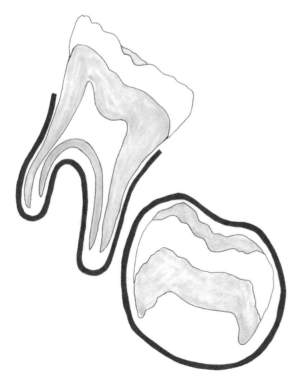

Fig. 11. The lamina dura (*shown in solid black*) is seen around erupted (the left) and unerupted (the right) teeth. It is equivalent to a cortex between dental structures and the surrounding mandibular or maxillary bone.

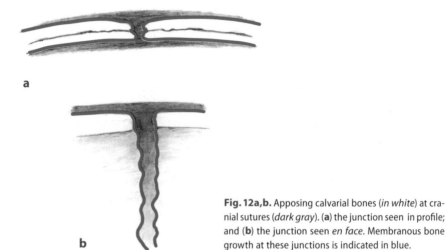

Fig. 12a,b. Apposing calvarial bones (*in white*) at cranial sutures (*dark gray*). (**a**) the junction seen in profile; and (**b**) the junction seen *en face*. Membranous bone growth at these junctions is indicated in blue.

tion crosses (and makes less dense) the lamina dura on the way to forming periapical abscess (which is in bone rather than soft tissue).

The flat bones of the calvarium, except at the skull base, are membranous growth bones. The dura mater acts as the internal surface periosteum. Periosteum-like tissue also lies along the outer (narrow) margins of these bones, along the sutures, creating membranous growth at those sites as well (Fig. 12). I presume the margins of intrasutural wormian bones similarly show membranous growth.

Some sources say that the terminal tufts of distal phalanges are formed in membrane. Some aspects of what happens to them are consistent with that designation (such as the relative sparing from enchondral growth destruction in frostbite); however, other aspects suggest that the margin is a zone of provisional calcification of an acrophysis (such as the occurrence of exostosis at the margin of a tuft). So far, I have not encountered a histologic study that confirms whether the margin is cortex or ZPC cartilage.

Vertebral Column and Other Apparently Non-Tubular Bones

The vertebral body grows by enchondral bone growth superiorly and inferiorly, with its front and sides like the shaft of a tubular bone (with periosteum or its equivalent) (Fig. 13). However, at birth, the enchondral physis extends downward in front of the vertebral body all the way to the vascular channel in its anterior middle. The superior and inferior endplates are actually zones of provisional calcification of physeal cartilage. The pedicles and other components of the posterior arch are analogues of long bones, with tubular enchondral bone growth and membranous periosteal growth. Therefore, they participate in all the vagaries of enchondral and membranous bone growth as tubular bones, with the exception that only a modified metaphy-

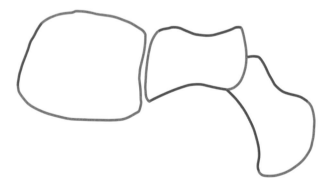

Fig. 13. Schematic representation of vertebral growth seen from the side. The endplates and posterior vertebral bodies grow enchondrally (*red*), while the increasing anterior body margin grows by membranous growth (*blue*). The arch elements grow in length enchondrally (*red*), while their shaft-equivalent width grows by membranous periosteum (*blue*).

seal collar exits adjacent to the enchondral ends of the pedicle and other arch elements. Similarly, iliac bones and scapula enchondral sites are analogous to the tubular bones with quite modified metaphyseal collar equivalents.

In osteoporotic conditions, the endplates, being ZPCs, are particularly conspicuous radiographically, in contrast to the adjacent demineralized bone. In contrast, in rickets with secondary hyperparathyroidism, the endplates, being uncalcified ZPCs, are noticeably inconspicuous/indistinct.

All epiphyseal dysplasias are to some extent spondyloepiphyseal dysplasias since the vertebral column has its sites of enchondral growth. However, the term spondyloepiphyseal dysplasia is reserved for certain ones with characteristic vertebral abnormalities. Similarly, all metaphyseal chondrodysplasias are to some extent spondylometaphyseal dysplasias.

For the vertebral column, one can expect enchondral disease to affect the appropriate sites while it can be anticipated that the other appropriate sites will be affected by membranous disease. Enchondral bone slowing in achondroplasia, for example, results in reduced height of vertebral bodies and is responsible for the severe spinal stenosis in the lower lumbar region, and occasionally in the upper cervical column. Whenever platyspondyly (generalized short height of vertebral bodies) occurs, one must surely check to insure that the dens is not too short, lest a tendency to atlantoaxial subluxation go unrecognized. In Marfan syndrome, with its acceleration of enchondral growth, the pedicles and laminae of the lumbar region are longer than normal, yielding a capacious lumbar spinal canal.

Many of the skull and facial bones are purely membranous in origin. Others, comprising the chondrocranium of the skull base and at least the condyles of the mandible, have enchondral growth as part of their pattern of maturation. Thus, in achondroplasia, the foramen magnum and jugular foramina of the skull base are small, with the latter sometimes responsible for hydrocephalus. Also, as a consequence of slowed growth of the chondrocranium, the superior semicircular canals are closer together in achondroplasia than in persons who grow normally (Fig. 14). Frontal bossing occurs in that dysplasia as anterior frontal bone membranous growth proceeds normally, while the skull base is enchondrally slowed and remains relatively small.

Tarsals, carpals, and sesamoids are all purely enchondral bones. The calcaneus is unusual in having its own apophysis posteriorly. The talus has its os trigonum centers, which behave a bit like apophyses, a bit like sesamoids.

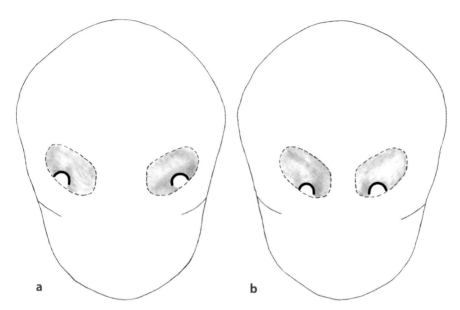

a   b

Fig. 14a,b. The superior semicircular canals (roofs indicated as *solid black curves*) in a normal (**a**) and in an achondroplastic (**b**) head, as seen projected through the orbits *(dotted lines)*. Because of the slowed enchondral growth at the skull base and central structures, those semicircular canals are closer to the midline in achondroplasia.

Stylohyoid ligaments are a fine example of ligaments that ossify. Indeed, after 18 months of age, up to 25% of children show some ossification, and with increasing frequency as children grow older. Since ossification is from a ligament, the stylohyoid may be considered membranous bone. In dysostosis multiplex, such as Hurler disease and other heteroglycanoses, the stylohyoid ligaments tend to ossify earlier, more frequently, and with wider ossification than in other children.

The acetabulum and glenoid are also sites that are affected by abnormalities of enchondral growth including, for example, osteoporosis and rickets. Moreover, the equivalent of cone epiphyses occurs due to impaired enchondral growth at the center of the acrophysis of the roof of the acetabulum (manifest as a "trident" acetabular roof) and the same can occur at the center of the glenoid of the scapula.

The ossicles of the middle ear, characteristic shape and all, are formed in membrane.

Frostbitten tubular bones become membranous-only whenever the physes and acrophyses at both ends of the bone (including of the epiphyses) have ceased growing.

5

Prenatal Development

Bone growth in the child is of course ongoing since the very onset of its prenatal development. Although I am not getting into all the embryology of prebone and the skeletal system, one should be aware that intrauterine bone growth is fundamentally the same as postnatal, in that it is either enchondral bone growth or membranous bone growth at each appropriate site.

Although weightbearing is not a factor affecting growth in utero, pressures from the relatively confined environment have effects, particularly when oligohydramnios is a factor. Genetics affects the initial appearance of concentrations of mesenchyme which form growth cartilage; and then, hox genes and other genetic and local induction factors affect connectivity and bone number and nature that will appear later on. Programmed fusion of bones may not occur until much later in childhood. Many ossification centers, both membranous and enchondral bone, appear prenatally. Knowledge that appearance of calcaneus is at about 23 weeks of gestation and talus at about 26 weeks and distal femur epiphysis at about 33 weeks may help in the estimation of maturation.

Intrauterine trauma, infection, and metabolic bone disease all affect bone growth locally or systematically. For example, one finds generalized delayed maturation of bone in prenatal hypothyroidism. Maternal vitamin-D deficiency is a cause of fetal rickets. On occasion, amniocentesis needles disturb a site of growth cartilage or periosteum. Intrauterine exposure to teratogens, including alcohol and dilantin, may affect overall growth (smallness for gestational age, for example) or certain skeletal features.

In twin-twin transfusion, the donor twin is typically small for gestational age, whereas the recipient is large. The donor twin may become "stuck" in the uterus and thus have decreased motion, which would lead to decreased skeletal development. I wonder if maturation is also delayed in the donor twin. Conjoined twins have a range of segmentation anomalies in the region where the twins are joined.

Poland syndactyly consists of a set of findings present at birth. The theory proposed by Dr. Josef Warkany is intriguing. The small to absent middle phalanges, with the ipsilateral poor development of the pectoral muscles, are proposed by Dr. Warkany to be caused by repeated intrauterine hitting of the ipsilateral chest with the clenched fist. To support his theory, Dr. Warkany cited cases of left-sided Poland syndrome with dextroposition of the heart, the suggestion being that the repeated pounding of the left anterior chest pushed the heart to the contralateral side. The associated soft tissue syndactyly, which seems like decreased apoptosis during development, might also be due to the effect of pressure upon the pounding wrist; however, that is more difficult to explain.

Babies may be born with fractures. Some are due to the traumatic delivery of a baby with normal bones; others are due to bone disease already present in utero. The classic multiple fractures at birth is in babies with osteogenesis imperfecta. Many fractures already show healing (indicating that they are at least 10 days old); some fractures have healed leaving bent broad-appearing bones. Some prenatally bent bones are susceptible to fracture as well. I have seen a newly born infant with curved femurs from Antley Bixler syndrome acquire a femur fracture in the absence of major trauma.

Tight intrauterine packing and positioning may well play a role in the development of clubfoot and of curvature of one or both tibias.

When in osteopetrosis, dense bone entails most of the marrow cavity at birth, which is sometimes the case, anemia will be severe. The metabolic segmental rickets-like abnormalities of hypophosphatasia have occasionally healed by birth, leaving normal metaphyseal appearance, but long bones are still curved, often with midshaft Bowdler spurs leading to skin dimples (Fig. 15). In the case of severe Jeune syndrome or in one of the short rib polydactyly syndromes, newborn babies with very short ribs may suffer respiratory death from being unable to breathe sufficiently once outside the uterus.

With recent stunning advances in prenatal skeletal imaging by ultrasound and MRI, many abnormalities of bone growth and skeletal function can now be diagnosed during the fetal period.

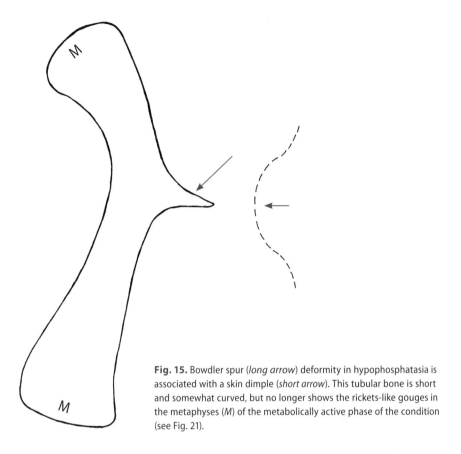

Fig. 15. Bowdler spur (*long arrow*) deformity in hypophosphatasia is associated with a skin dimple (*short arrow*). This tubular bone is short and somewhat curved, but no longer shows the rickets-like gouges in the metaphyses (*M*) of the metabolically active phase of the condition (see Fig. 21).

6

Exostoses and Enchondromas

An exostosis, whether solitary or part of multiple exostoses (a dysplasia, also known as osteochondromatosis), grows enchondrally from a misdirected cartilaginous cap. That cap closely resembles a conventional growth plate (Fig. 16). To emphasize that resemblance, I call the growth plate of the cartilage cap, "*paraphysis*" [para = alongside, from the Greek]. This paraphysis is subject to all the vagaries of the physis and acrophysis in cases of generalized abnormality. If ever you see a subject with exostosis who has rickets, I predict the loss of its ZPC and I would appreciate seeing the example. Growth of the exostosis from its paraphysis continues until the end of enchondral growth in adolescence.

Trevor disease, also called dysplasia epiphysealis hemimelica, represents exostoses of secondary growth centers. As they are arising from a purely enchondral bony part, they may not have a well-formed growth plate at the margin, but the growth is indeed from cartilage, a sort of acroparaphysis.

Exostoses can arise wherever a growth plate can go "astray" in a direction other than what is normal. Even the paraphysis growth plate of an exostosis can go astray, causing the development of an exostosis of an exostosis. Acrophyses can have their own acroexostoses, either in the form of Trevor disease or along the nonepiphyseal shaft site of a small tubular bone. When an acroexostosis arises adjacent to a terminal tuft of a finger or toe phalanx, it supports the notion that the distal tuft margin is an acrophyseal zone of provisional calcification rather than membranous thin cortex.

Each exostosis uses up longitudinal growth potential, i.e., the more and the larger the exostosis of a bone, the less the bone reaches its otherwise programmed growth potential. This principle is most graphically seen with paired tubular bones; the one with more exostoses has greater decrease in length potential, leaving the other paired bone to become bowed (Fig. 17).

The aleatoric [chance-distribution] dysplasia of multiple enchondromas is called Ollier disease. Whatever goes genetically awry in the multiple cartilage persistence in the metaphyses causing enchondromas leads to a lack of ossification, presumably from the withholding of vascularity. It is then ironic that Maffucci syndrome adds multiple hemangiomas of soft tissues, which are vascular lesions. The most unfortunate part of Maffucci syndrome is the high incidence of malignant degeneration of lesions (tumors of at least in part cartilaginous histology).

Uncommonly, a single patient can show a hybrid of both enchondromas and exostoses.

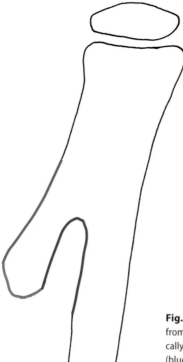

Fig. 16. An exostosis on a stalk grows in length enchondrally from a paraphysis (*red*) that closely resembles a physis histologically; while its sides form by membranous periosteal growth (blue) that blends into the cortex of the host bone. Sessile exostoses grow similarly, but are broader rather than stalked.

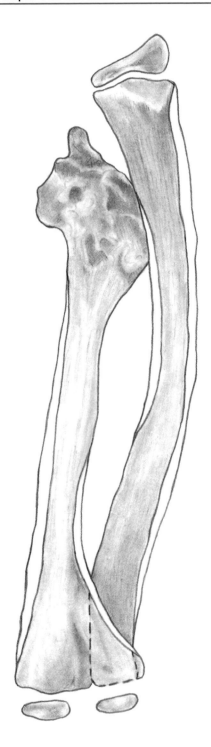

Fig. 17. The larger the exostoses, the more that longitudinal growth is diverted from its adjacent physes. Thus, this ulna with large exostoses is shorter than its companion radius that lacks large exostoses.

7

Metabolic Bone Disease

Whatever effect metabolic bone disease has on physeal growth is also manifest at acrophyseal sites; whatever effect it has on membranous bone growth will affect all membranous sites including flat bones as well as tubular bone shafts.

Most variations from the norm caused by metabolic abnormality are systematic and symmetric, with some exceptions. For example, the fractures that occur with weakened bones are not systematic, being caused, instead, by a combination of chance and the activity of the child. Some conditions that manifest periosteal reaction also have a nonsystematic distribution (for example, hypervitaminosis A).

In **rickets**, every zone of provisional calcification [ZPC] is uncalcified (Fig. 18). The cartilage of each physis and acrophysis, which should normally be calcified, isn't calcified. As a result unossified cartilage builds up. Thus, the soft tissue space between epiphyses and metaphyses is wider than normal; epiphyses and their equivalents tend to be unsharp in their margins (due to the lack of ZPC); and bone age does not advance (the growth remains cartilaginous and thus it is not radiographically visible); the region of the metaphyseal collar will not have bone within the region bounded by the bone bark, and therefore, the metaphyseal collar is "lost" since no longer is ossified bone bordered by the collar (Fig. 19). I have given a name to this not-yet-ossified growth material, which ought to be bone and yet isn't. I call it **pseudophysis**. With the exception of rickets due to phosphate loss from kidneys, secondary hyperparathyroidism soon occurs. The distal ulna early in childhood is often normally concave at its distal ossified margin. Consequently, it should not be considered a diagnostic feature of rickets. Other bone ends eventually seem cupped in rickets, i.e., metaphyseal membranous bone growth at the collar continues transversely, making the bone end look broad (especially the anterior rib ends, appearing as the "rachitic rosary"). Moreover, continued bone bark ossification makes the bone ends in rickets look frayed or jagged. Seeing the pattern of the early healing of rickets (Fig. 20), when at first only the ZPC reappears, helps explain what is invisible on radiograph in active rickets (see Fig. 18).

Rickets is a condition of the growing child. "No growth" means "no rickets" (until growth resumes). Example: A child with lack of growth secondary to hypothyroidism from cystinosis, with cystine deposits in the thyroid; when thyroid hormone was replaced, the child began to grow and rickets became manifest. A child with severe renal osteodystrophy was not growing. Following renal transplantation, rapid resumption of growth occurred and rickets was evident until treated. I refer to a condition in which a child has all the potential for rickets but is not growing, as being *"pre-rickets."* Many severely undernourished children may well be in a pre-rickets state.

Hypophosphatasia: has several interesting characteristics on imaging. Most notably, it resembles rickets in a spatially incomplete fashion (Fig. 21). The zones of unmineralized cartilage persisting into metaphysis are occasionally seen at the margins of enchondral secondary growth centers, persisting into bone of the center which is otherwise ossified (Fig. 21).

The pattern of bone growth abnormality in *aluminum intoxication* is the same as in rickets. I would thus consider this to be a form of rickets. Bone changes can be severe and can resolve somewhat more slowly than conventional nutritional rickets.

In children, a key to recognizing *osteoporosis* on radiographs is the *cartilage zone of provisional calcification*, which maintains its usual density, while the bone adjacent to it becomes less dense than normal (see Fig. 22). As a result, the ZPC becomes quite conspicuous as a thin, dense line at all sites of enchondral growth; as opposed to rickets, in which the ZPC doesn't calcify and so is much less conspicuous. If a child were to have both osteoporosis and rickets, the ZPC would also fail to be visible; hence, eliminating this osteoporotic recognition method.

The most frequent cause of osteoporosis in childhood, both in hospital and outpatient practice, is disuse osteoporosis, due to orthopaedic immobilization. Osteoporosis in the immobilized region is almost invariable. When

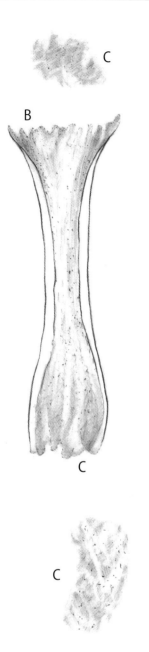

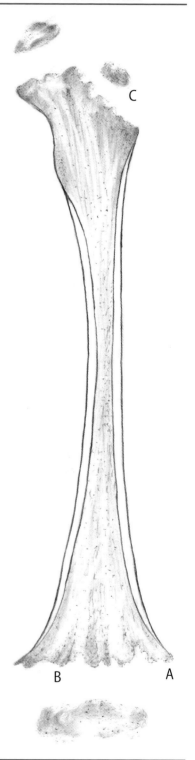

Fig. 18. Schematic representation of rickets. Metaphyseal collars are not seen (*A*), and zones of provisional calcification are not calcified at physes (*B*) or at acrophyses (*C*). These unmineralized areas begin to return upon successful treatment, beginning with the ZPCs (see Fig. 20).

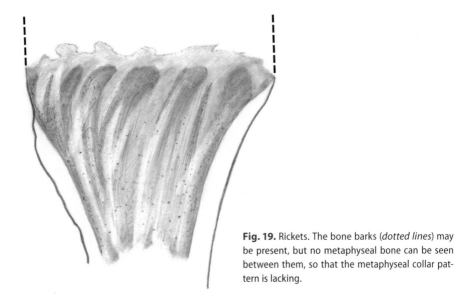

Fig. 19. Rickets. The bone barks (*dotted lines*) may be present, but no metaphyseal bone can be seen between them, so that the metaphyseal collar pattern is lacking.

a child starts running again after a leg or foot cast has been removed, insufficiency or stress fractures through the demineralized bone are quite common. This is recognizable after 10 days by endosteal callus in tarsal bones or periosteal reaction along tubular bones. The fracture callus, like the ZPC, is recognized as being more dense than the osteoporotic bone. With increased activity, once the cast has been removed and the fractures have healed, this form of osteoporosis is reversed.

Osteoporosis in childhood may be idiopathic (at least until such time as a cause has been determined in the individual or by advances in pediatric science, not yet achieved). Other causes include osteoporosis due to the use of steroids (intrinsic or extrinsic, especially in high doses), certain other drugs that may modify the body's growth economy, lack of muscular activity, weightlessness (OK, to date, no children have yet been sent into space), juvenile idiopathic arthritis (that's still JRA in parts of the USA) even when not yet treated, and leukemia. Historically, a frequent cause of childhood osteoporosis was *scurvy*. Many of the classic radiographic findings of scurvy, even those with special names, are really those of osteoporosis. In addition, the tendency to epiphyseolysis is high in active children with active scurvy, notably the slipped distal femoral epiphysis.

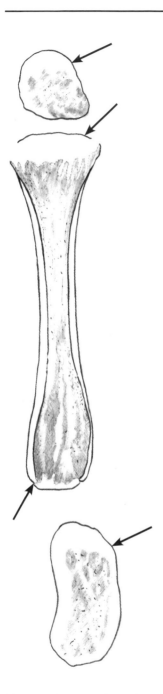
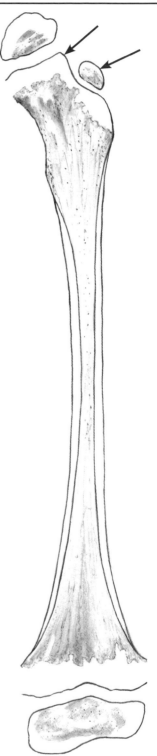

Fig. 20. Early recovery from rickets. The zones of provisional calcification (some indicated by arrows) are the first previously unmineralized structures to reappear (compare Fig. 18, active rickets).

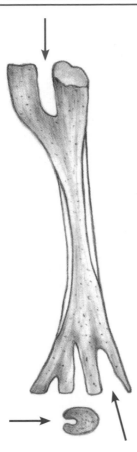

Fig. 21. Metabolically active hypophosphatasia of a tubular bone (and its epiphysis). Arrows indicate some of the gouges (zones) of uncalcified metaphysis (or of metaphyseal equivalent in the growth center). These gouges are interspersed with normally mineralized areas.

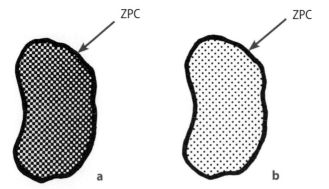

Fig. 22a,b. Compared to normally dense bones in childhood (**a**), where the zone of provisional calcification (arrow) is moderately well distinguishable from bone, the osteoporotic bones (**b**) show a far more conspicuous (normally dense) cartilage zone of provisional calcification (*arrow*) interfacing with less dense less mineralized bone.

Hyperparathyroidism seems most frequent as a secondary metabolic/ endocrine response to rickets. Primary hyperparathyroidism, due to parathyroid adenoma or other autonomous hyperfunction of the parathyroid gland(s), is less common. The radiographic features of hyperparathyroidism are all different from osteoporosis, which is the other major cause of generalized demineralization of bone in children. Perhaps the most basic is the increased tunneling = "washing out" = loss of definition of cortex in hyperparathyroidism (Fig. 23). In osteoporosis, cortex eventually is thinned, but in hyperparathyroidism it loses the solidness of definition. Equivalent and important diagnostic features of hyperparathyroidism are loss of the lamina dura around erupted and unerupted teeth (Fig. 24), and a salt-and-pepper look to calvarial bones (increased tunneling seen *en face*). Increased coarseness of trabeculae in metaphyses and diaphyseal bone is another recognizable feature, as is easy fracturability through these affected bones. The trabecular structure of growth centers within their ZPC (or within the purported site of the presumed ZPC when rickets is present) is also coarse

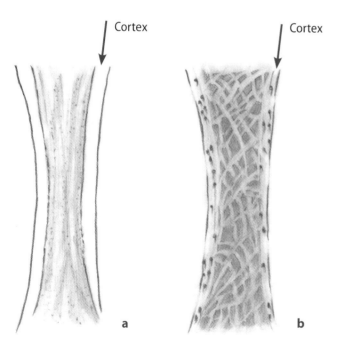

Fig. 23a,b. Compared to normal cortex (**a**), in hyperparathyroidism (**b**) cortices are more tunneled and appear washed-out. Within the medullary portion of bones with hyperparathyroidism, trabeculae appear fewer and more prominent than normal.

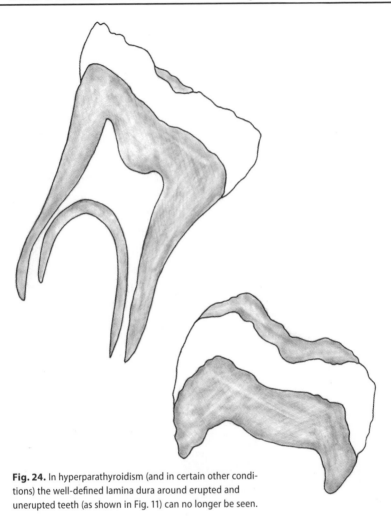

Fig. 24. In hyperparathyroidism (and in certain other conditions) the well-defined lamina dura around erupted and unerupted teeth (as shown in Fig. 11) can no longer be seen.

in hyperparathyroidism. A less common feature today is the brown tumor of hyperparathyroidism (for those who remember the cartoon-in-a-cartoon character, Fearless Fosdick, the lucencies of brown tumors may resemble the bullet holes through the clothes and body of that intrepid detective; I call it the Fearless Fosdick sign). Brown tumors are reactive tumor-like zones full of many giant cells and other non-bone matter. The radiographic pattern of primary and secondary hyperparathyroidism is the same, except of course when the findings of rickets are seen in the secondary form.

In *"heavy metal" poisoning*, usually due to lead intoxication, but also, especially in years gone by, to bismuth transplacental intoxication, bone created

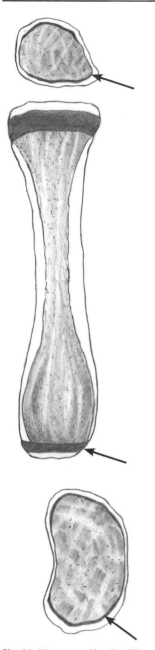

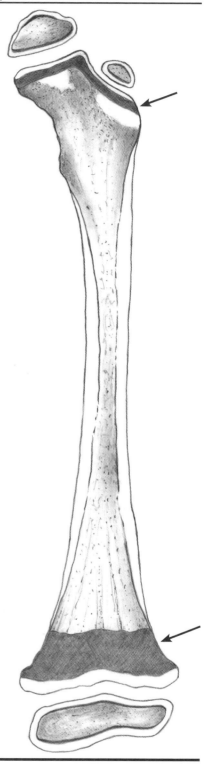

Fig. 25. "Heavy metal" or "lead" lines, shown here as dense bands, including in growth centers, some indicated by arrows. As with lucent "leukemic" lines (see Fig. 26), they nearly parallel the zones of provisional calcification at physes and acrophyses. The width of the bands are proportional to the rates of enchondral growth at each site.

at every physis and acrophysis is laid down more tightly packed than normal, and then yields a denser band than normal bone as growth proceeds, roughly paralleling the physis or acrophysis from whence it came (Fig. 25). The more rapid the site of enchondral growth, the further the line/band will be from the physis or acrophysis once normal growth resumes. If a child presents with encephalopathy, it's best to assume that lead poisoning is the cause of any lead lines. Otherwise, dense lines/bands in the metaphyseal regions may also be physiologic or due to minor illness or other adverse events of childhood, on the way to becoming growth arrest/recovery lines. However, poisoning due to insecticides and other industrial products, and the jolt from having been injected with powerful drugs such as chemotherapeutic agents, also result in radiodense lines of tightly packed bone, paralleling physes and acrophyses.

As opposed to the dense lines/bands of heavy metals and other poisonings, *"leukemic" lines*, or bands, are more lucent than normal neighboring bone as well as the ZPC (Fig. 26). Whenever the body "economy" is impaired by major stress, it seems that bone created enchondrally during that period becomes less dense than it would otherwise be (with the exception of lead and similar poisoning, which is more dense than normal). The most frequent cause of so-called leukemic lines is *birth*. Thus, almost all newborns, after about 10 days of age, show lucent metaphyseal bands associated with the "stress" of adjusting to extrauterine life. The ZPC remains of normal density. The equivalent pattern seen in the vertebral column of infants after 10 days is the "bone-in-bone" pattern: the vertebral end plates, which are ZPCs, maintain normal density and the prenatal bone is of "normal" bone density; however, postnatal bone in-between is relatively demineralized. Consequently, the normal prenatal bone appears as apparently dense bone within a bone. The same pattern appears in such enchondral bone centers as calcaneus and talus. Later in the first year of life, those metaphyseal lucent bands are no longer seen. If a newborn less than 10 days of age already shows lucent bands, that is a sign of intrauterine stress. This is the nonspecific reason why some babies born with syphilis have the lucent bands at birth, which should be evident on chest images. There is no need for a bone survey in neonatal syphilis until local signs and symptoms suggest local syphilic bone disease. One more reason for well-defined "leukemic" lucent metaphyseal bands at birth is magnesium compounds given to the mother to delay the onset of labor when premature delivery is a concern. When a child is several years of age, leukemic

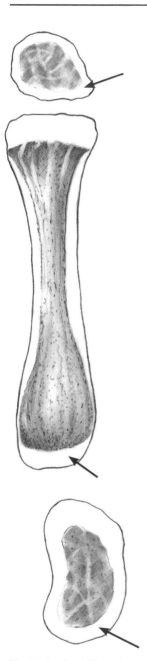

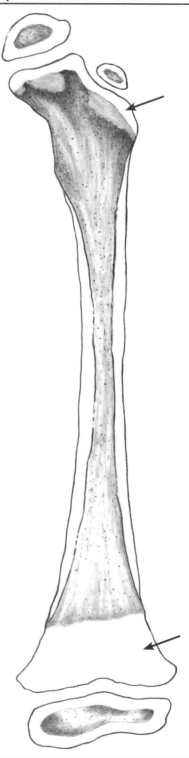

Fig. 26. "Leukemic" lines, shown here as the lucent bands, including in growth centers, some indicated with arrows. As with "lead" lines (see Fig. 25), they nearly parallel the zones of provisional calcification at physes and acrophyses. The width of the bands are proportional to the rates of enchondral growth at each site.

lines in the proximal humerus on a chest radiograph may indeed be the first radiographic feature leading to a diagnosis of leukemia. However, any major illness or long period of hospitalization often yields similar demineralized metaphyseal bands.

Interestingly in cases of *vitamin-D overdose*, either lucent or dense bands can appear in metaphyses. Your choice of explanation.

Beyond the excessive function of the parathyroids discussed above, a variety of other endocrine diseases affect bone growth. *Growth hormone deficiency,* or (in Laron disease, lack of normal response to growth hormone), gives proportional delay in bone maturation and growth. However, bones have normal shape, although stature is short. *Hypothyroidism* also has delayed bone age and growth, but unlike growth hormone deficiency, the bones do not have normal shape. Both epiphyseal irregularity of shape and density, and later metaphyseal irregularity of shape and density, each resembling dysplasia, occur. In *hypogonadism*, such as low or absent estrogen, that component of bone maturation which leads to closure of physes near the end of growth is impaired, so that bones may continue to grow past the normal time and become increasingly long. One cause of low estrogen in girls is a very high level of sports performance, which would give a vicious circle of sorts. The delay in the ending of longitudinal growth makes the individual tall, which has an advantage in sports such as basketball, so that the high physical activity level persists, as does the low estrogen. Too much steroid from the overfunction of the *adrenals* by themselves or from tumor, or, in Nelson syndrome, from too much positive signal from the pituitary via ACTH, will yield osteoporosis.

Physiologic periosteal reaction from normal rapid growth in infancy has been shown by Volberg and colleagues (by analogy) in puppies [Volberg FM Jr, Whalen JP, Krook L, Winchester P. Lamellated periosteal reactions: a radiologic and histologic investigation. AJR Am J Roentgenol. 1977, 128:85-7.] and by Shopfner and his technologists with both sick and well babies [Shopfner CE. Periosteal bone growth in normal infants. A preliminary report. Am J Roentgenol Radium Ther Nucl Med. 1966, 97:154-63]. Periosteal reaction is seen normally (physiologically) beginning from about one to six months of age in humans and at an equivalent age in puppies, and lasting several months, until joining the cortex itself. This periosteal reaction is symmetric along long bones and should not be confused with pathologic periosteal reaction. I have seen a case of growth hormone-producing tumor of the pituitary much later in childhood that induced such a rapid spurt of growth that similar periosteal reaction was seen along the small tubular bones on a bone age image.

The distribution of periosteal reaction in *hypervitaminosis A* is unusual, and therefore if recognized can speed the diagnosis of that condition. The reaction is typically along the ulnas, the fibulas, and the fifth metatarsals (I don't know why. Do you?). Often pseudotumor cerebri is associated, so look for widened cranial sutures.

High dose prostaglandin E (E1 or E2), typically given for weeks to months to keep an infant's patent ductus arteriosus open, has as a frequent effect periosteal reaction along long bones, ribs and mandible, with associated redness, soft tissue swelling, and pain. These findings subside when the drug is discontinued. Other effects of prostaglandin E include narrowing of the stomach antrum from focal foveal hyperplasia.

Because infantile cortical hyperostosis, widely known as *Caffey disease*, behaves clinically and radiographically like high-dose prostaglandin E, it can be considered among endocrine diseases. However, it may (perhaps) be viral in origin and can run in families. If the periosteal reaction is present at birth, clearly the onset was prenatal. Each pregnancy with an at-birth Caffey disease infant that has the degree of amniotic fluid recorded, has had polyhydramnios; presumably the fetus does not normally swallow fluid because of mandible pain from the condition.

The vigorous periosteal reaction along tubular bones of the feet, as well as other tubular bones in *mother-of-pearl worker disease* of Central Europe, behaves as a reaction to inhalation of toxic dust. Similarly, *hypertrophic pulmonary osteoarthropathy* seems a reactive response to disturbance in the parts of the body served by the vagus nerve, namely the chest and liver. In children, this complication in my experience is most likely to occur with severe cystic fibrosis (affecting the lungs and often the liver); I have also seen it associated with actinomycosis of the right lung and chest wall.

Intrauterine exposure to toxins can affect bone growth systematically by causing intrauterine growth retardation, but it may also have more specific manifestations such as those from exposure to dilantin or alcohol. Intrauterine exposure to warfanin (Coumadin) taken by the mother is one of the causes of multiple stippled epiphyses. I have seen this manifestation especially in the hindfoot.

Child abuse can also be considered as a "*metabolic*" disease. Neglect, for example, is a metabolic-like condition, given the name deprivational dwarfism (either emotional or nutritional deprivation) with poor growth and delayed bone age as manifestations. On presentation, the child may also have a greatly dilated stomach. Pancreatic injury from abuse may lead to infarctions of bone. Abuse fractures may simulate those seen in osteoporosis, but are secondary to abnormal trauma rather than abnormal bone. One should always also consider non-abuse causes of the fractures, including osteogenesis imperfecta. Menkes syndrome (in boys), and leukemia.

8 Dysplasias and Dysostoses

Several dichotomies are fundamental in consideration of the patterns of abnormal growth known as dysplasias and dysostoses: *systematic vs. aleatoric* [i.e., chance distribution of abnormalities] conditions; *slowed vs. accelerated growth* (vs. growth otherwise disordered); and *enchondral vs. membranous growth abnormality* (with the special case of perichondral metaphyseal collar abnormality). The current explosion of genetic knowledge is pertinent to our discussion but will only be included selectively. Thus, allelic (or near allelic) genetic changes may cause quite dissimilar manifestations or quite similar manifestations that have been grouped into families of disorders.

Less systematic than dysplasias are the dysostoses, disorders of several aspects of growth that are, however, not systematic, but yet a regular set of recognized malformations. Cleidocranial dysplasia/dysostosis, with its scattered findings of skull, clavicle, pubic symphysis, vertebral bodies, and tubular bones of the hands and feet, is considered a dysplasia by some experts and a dysostosis by others.

Achondroplasia is the prototype of systematic slowed-growth enchondral dysplasia. With several related dysplasias which share a genetic locus, it forms a family of dysplasias. Thanatophoric dysplasia is a more severe member of the achondroplasia family; hypochondroplasia is a less severe member.

Because membranous growth is normal, while enchondral growth is slowed, in achondroplasia, tubular bones look "wide", although they are actually of normal width, while the length is decreased (Fig. 27). Similar disproportionate growth gives abnormal shape to flat bones, such as ilium, and in the

Fig. 27. Achondroplasia, indicating schematically some of the consequences of slowed enchondral growth. Compared to normal, the tubular bones are shorter and appear broader (because membranous growth in width is normal), metaphyseal medial and lateral margins are more concave (shorter radius of curvature), and physes tend to form cone [middle indentation] configurations.

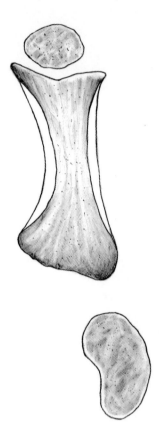
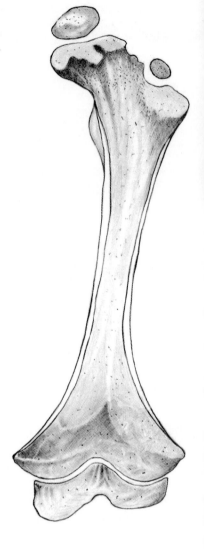

vertebral arches, which, being shortened, give a narrow spinal canal (Fig. 28). The longitudinal length of the metaphyseal collar is shorter than normal in achondroplasia (at the distal radius and ulna being 1mm or less, rather than the usual 1-3 mm; Fig. 29). Because of the decreased enchondral:membranous bone growth ratio, the outer and inner margins of metaphyses (the parts where periosteum lies) are more concave (shorter radius of curvature) than normal. Because of that decreased ratio, the calvarium seems to overgrow

Fig. 28. Achondroplasia: frontal view schema of lumbar vertebrae. The transverse distance between pedicles at each level decreases from L1 through L5, whereas in normal subjects, it increases.

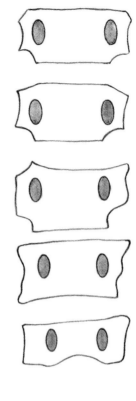

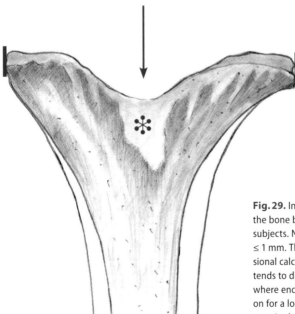

Fig. 29. In achondroplasia, the length of the bone bark (in *blue*) is less than normal subjects. Normal: 1–3 mm; achondroplasia ≤ 1 mm. The metaphyseal/zone of provisional calcification contour at the physis tends to dip in the central portion *(arrow)* … where enchondral slowing has been going on for a longer time. "✳" marks cartilage rests in the metaphysis, frequently occurring in achondroplasia.

compared to the chondrocranium base, causing frontal bossing (convex forward frontal bone, looks like *umbo*, the boss of a shield).

The *dolichostenomelias* are *dysplasias* with systematic acceleration of enchondral growth with normal rate of membranous growth; the prototype is **Marfan syndrome**. The other most prominent diagnosis is **homocystinuria**. Both have similar rhizomelic lengthening. The metaphyseal/metadiaphyseal margins at the knees and other ends of long bones are less concave (i.e., straighter) than normal (Fig. 30), especially when compared to the rhizomelic shortening disorders such as achondroplasia.

The prototype of a membranous growth bone dysplasia is **osteogenesis imperfecta**, with its osteoporotic thin cortices and easy fracturability (as well as the tell-tale multiple wormian intrasutural bones of the cranium, a characteristic it shares with multiple other conditions). OI is a condition of decreased membranous growth; the disease most typical of increased membranous bone growth is **Engelmann disease**, also called progressive diaphyseal dysplasia, in which diaphyseal cortex is thickened from excessive membranous growth.

The best known aleatoric dysplasias, multiple exostosis and multiple enchondromas, are discussed in Chapter 6.

In *metatropic dysplasia*, not only do we see the effects of enchondral slowing, but also the metaphyseal collar does not seem to have as tight a control as usual on the transverse widening of the metaphysis and adjoining physis. The result is a tubular bone shape which resembles either a dumbbell or a diabolo, more so than in the classic enchondral slowing entity of achondroplasia (Fig. 31). Thus metatropic dysplasia shares both enchondral slowing and the weakening of one aspect of membranous growth.

As discussed elsewhere, the aleatoric dysplasia, multiple stippled epiphyses, eventually turns into multiple epiphyseal dysplasias.

OSMED and **Kniest** disease are the least uncommon of the megaepiphyseal dysplasias. OSMED is **O**tospondylo**m**ega**e**piphyseal **d**ysplasia. Kniest disease has earlier and greater than normal enlargement of epiphyseal centers except for the femoral heads. The femoral heads are enlarged (and deformed) in cartilage but the ossification is delayed.

Many other genetic dysplasias and dysostoses are encountered, with varying degrees of rarity. The art of their radiographic recognition and classification must be learned, along with knowledge of where to go for help to see if a given example falls into a known category.

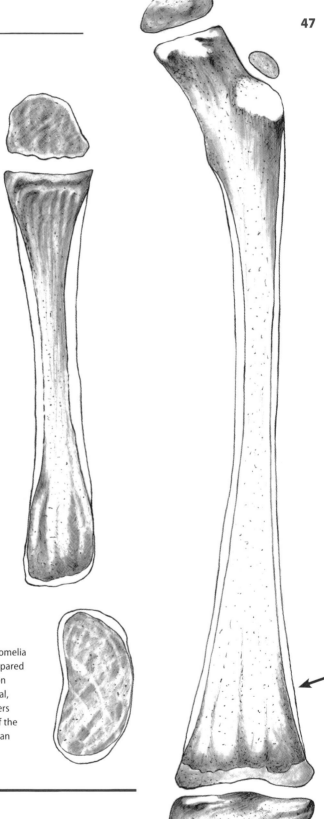

Fig. 30. Marfan syndrome dolichostenomelia schematic (printed reduced in size compared to the normal, say Fig. 1, so that it fits on page). The shafts are longer than normal, enchondral maturation at growth centers may be accelerated, and the margins of the metaphyses (*arrow*) are less concave than normal.

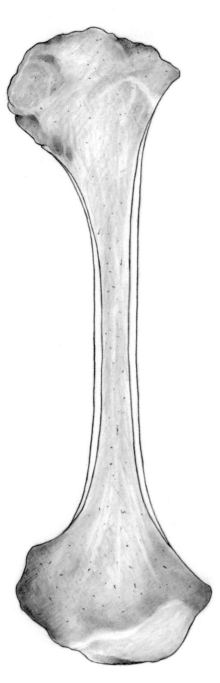

Fig. 31. Metatropic dysplasia long bone shaft schematic. Not only are bones short with more concave metaphyseal edges, (as in, say, achondroplasia), but also the metaphyses are even wider transversely (lack of restraint by metaphyseal collar?), giving an overall "dumbbell" shape.

9 Connectedness, Hox Genes

The effects on growth of abnormalities of segmentation or of number can be deduced from the abnormality itself, although some associations may be subtle and need to be learned (or looked up) for a complete evaluation. If, for example, a finger or toe is duplicated, the result on growth is different if equal duplication of all phalanges occurs, or if instead, one of the duplicated rays is smaller than the other, or a growth plate of one or both is incomplete, causing angular growth in a "wrong" direction of one or both rays.

In the **domed talus (ball-in-socket) ankle** deformity, the customarily flat upper bony margin of the talus (on the frontal radiograph, for example) is convex upwards and the lower margins of tibia and fibula articulating with it are abnormally concave, reflecting the same difference in shape, hence a ball-in-socket (Fig. 32). With domed talus, an association with tarsal coalition is present in at least half of the examples. The coalitions are not generally evident on plain images until the second decade of life, although the cartilaginous fusion can be detected sooner by MRI and sometimes ultrasound imaging. Interestingly, if tarsal bones are surgically fused, such as by stapling, during development, the result often is also a ball-in-socket ankle and domed talus. Other frequent associations with domed talus are short fibula (or even fibular hemimelia; i.e., absent fibula), short tibia with absence or hypoplasia of the proximal tibial spines, and short femur, sometimes including proximal focal femoral dysplasia. Tarsal centers may show small size or delayed development in infancy, which may allow one to predict that the domed talus and perhaps associated tarsal coalition will occur as the child develops.

The number of ribs and vertebrae at each level are under the control of *hox genes*. We found only about 85% of individuals to have the classic division of seven cervical vertebral bodies, 12 rib-bearing thoracic vertebral levels, and five lumbar levels. Others have cervical ribs, 12 or 13 rib pairs, only four lumbar bodies, transitional levels that have lumbar character on one side and sacral on the other, and various asymmetric versions of the above, such as 11 ribs on one side and 12 on the other.

Similar homeotic variation occurs in the limbs, cranium, and face – polydactyly and syndactyly are among the more common, as are transverse fusion of carpal bones. Absorption of the posterior arch of C1 into the occiput is yet another such variation.

VATER: One of the commonest of the *V* (= vertebral) findings in the VATER/VACTERL association is variation from normal in the number of rib-bearing vertebrae, i.e., other than 12 rib pairs. Otherwise stated, perhaps over half of individuals with esophageal atresia have other than 12 rib pairs (for example, one or two 13th ribs or one or two sides with only 11 ribs). For completeness, *A* = *A*nal malformation, such as imperforation; *C* = *C*ardiac malformation; *TE* = *T*racheo *E*sophageal, fistulas and atresias; *R* = *R*enal (or *R*adial); and *L* = *L*imb (which some incorporate into R for Radial)

An anteriorly *forked rib* is a fairly common and sometimes confusing anomaly of segmentation, presumably a hox gene effect, i.e., a posterior rib splits into two anterior ribs. Another variation is merely an anterior widening of a rib without splitting into two. Similar forking segmentation anomalies are occasionally seen in long bones and I have seen it once at a lateral clavicle. Generally, only one end of the split tubular bone articulates with the apposing bone (with ribs, each anterior end joins its cartilage, which, for all but the lower rib, then articulates with the sternum).

The unfortunate malformation known as *sirenomelia* is basically one in which only one midline lower extremity has formed. It may have two complete sets of lower extremity bones, close together, in parallel, within a single soft tissue structure, but more classically, a single femur only articulates with a tibia and/or fibula, and then ankle and foot bones. The pubic symphysis is fused or more narrow than normal, with a small pelvis. The bladder and other cloacal structures may be tiny or absent and as a result, no functioning kidneys are formed (and therefore, oligohydramnios is present in utero).

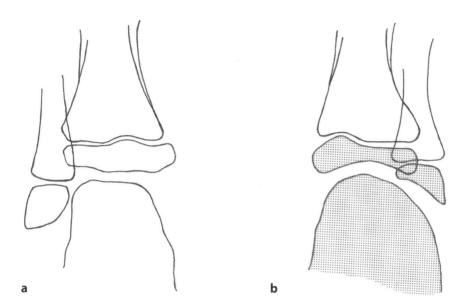

Fig. 32a,b. Compared to normal (**a**), the domed talus complex (**b**) has a convex proximal talus on frontal view, the "ball," which fits into its "socket," the abnormally concave lower margins of the distal epiphyses of tibia and fibula.

10 Local Impairment or Speeding of Enchondral Growth

Generalized impairment of bone growth, from dysplasia, metabolic bone disease, illness/malnutrition, or hormone dysfunction, is both generalized and systematic in slowing growth proportionate to the normal rates of enchondral growth. In this chapter, we consider local impairment. If, for example, growth is slowed in one lower extremity and not the other, unequal leg lengths would lead to a limp. Similarly, local increase in growth leads to unequal length.

Frostbite effects on growth of distal fingers (or toes) are quite well known. But did you know that the acrophyses of the involved phalanges may also be impaired? Indeed they are, resulting in termination of growth or of portions of growth at nonepiphyseal ends of involved phalanges (Fig. 33). Interestingly, terminal tufts do not seem to be impaired (which is a factor favoring membranous rather than enchondral growth at those tufts). Those phalanges whose physes are most affected are short in association with fusion of the physes. The phalanges of the thumb are often, but not always, spared, presumably because of relative protection of the thumb curled into the fist or palm at the time of the cold injury. Heat or electric injury to the distal fingers eventually yields similar patterns of early fusion and shortening (although in the near term, following the accident, maturation may be accelerated). Similar enchondral damage and slowing or elimination occurs, but is different in the location of affected bones, in *Kashin Beck disease* (Fig. 34), as well as from infection secondary to ratbite. Kashin Beck disease is mysterious but has affected hundred of thousands of individuals, especially in China and Tibet.

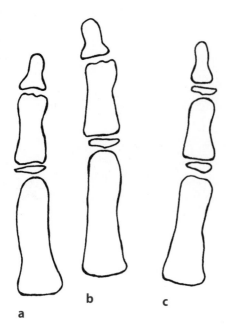

Fig. 33. Schematic of three finger phalanges in a case of frostbite. Note that distal phalanges (**a**) and (**b**) are short compared to the unaffected phalanx (**c**), and the physes of distal phalanges (**a**) and (**b**) have fused. Moreover, the head of middle phalanges (**a**) and (**b**) are irregular, due to acrophyseal enchondral damage from the frostbite cold episode.

   Trauma may result in growth changes in at least three ways: the vascularity of healing of fractures causing acceleration of enchondral growth; damage to the zone of resting cartilage of enchondral growth plates causing impairment of growth, and bridging of bone across physis; causing tethering of growth.

   Whenever the zone of resting cartilage of a growth plate is lost, no further cartilage forms from that plate. If resting cartilage of part of a plate is lost, that part of the growth potential is lost, for example central loss causes cone epiphysis (Fig. 35); asymmetric loss of part of a growth plate causes asymmetric loss of growth.

   If growth plate loss/tethering is asymmetric, then growth is "turned" (Fig. 36). The analogy may be made to a column of marching persons, which turns when a portion of the lead marchers stays in place while those next to them continue walking. Medial tethering will cause varus; lateral tethering will cause valgus; and anterior, posterior or other tethering causes the expected similar result.

   Cone epiphysis is usually a description of small tubular bone epiphyseal ends, but the same events give the same appearance at epiphyses of long tubular bones. A central portion of growth plate is slowed or more often has lost its growth (loss of the zone of resting cartilage) with a central bony bridge

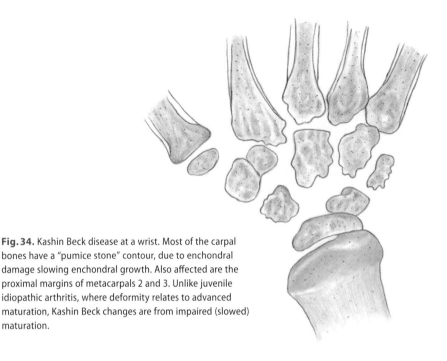

Fig. 34. Kashin Beck disease at a wrist. Most of the carpal bones have a "pumice stone" contour, due to enchondral damage slowing enchondral growth. Also affected are the proximal margins of metacarpals 2 and 3. Unlike juvenile idiopathic arthritis, where deformity relates to advanced maturation, Kashin Beck changes are from impaired (slowed) maturation.

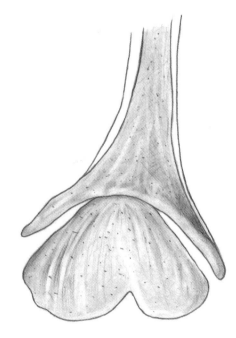

Fig. 35. Schematic of a cone-shaped epiphysis complex. Growth has been terminated in the older, central part of the physis, tethering further local growth; the metaphyseal margin toward the epiphysis is concave; and the epiphysis "sinks in" to this concavity, getting the shape of a cone. The medial and lateral metaphyseal margins tend also to be more concave than normal because of the net slowed enchondral growth.

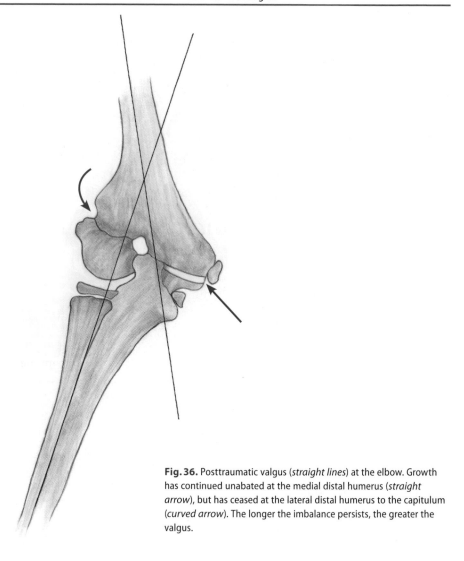

Fig. 36. Posttraumatic valgus (*straight lines*) at the elbow. Growth has continued unabated at the medial distal humerus (*straight arrow*), but has ceased at the lateral distal humerus to the capitulum (*curved arrow*). The longer the imbalance persists, the greater the valgus.

from metaphysis to epiphysis. As a result of continued growth of newer, more peripheral parts of the physis, the epiphysis seems to sink into the metaphysis as a cone-like configuration. As transverse widening continues of the viable less central growth plate, new enchondral growth is progressively further toward the peripheral end of the bone, compared to the central tether (see Fig. 35).

The so-called trident acetabular roof is of the same origin as the cone epiphysis, with deformity of that acetabular roof (or equivalently, the glenoid of the shoulder) as a result of central tethered growth.

The physeal ossified "*hyphen*" does not tether or impair growth. Over 50% of children will show one or more thin calcified or ossified lines perpendicular (or obliquely nearly perpendicular) to the physis of distal radius or ulna (Fig. 37). Those lines, which we term hyphens for want of a better name, once they appear, continue to be present throughout the years of growth. If you look carefully, you typically can see a continuation of the hyphen as a thin line extending a variable distance into the shaft of the involved bone, increasingly long as childhood growth proceeds. Whatever it is, it does not seem to tether the physis or retard growth in any way. Similar hyphens are occasionally seen at the distal tibia or fibula or even other physes. Incidentally, hyphens at the wrist have also been seen in monkeys. I have seen hyphens that were still present in rickets even when the metaphyseal collar bone was otherwise unossified.

Any higher than normal vascularity in a site of enchondral growth during childhood leads to acceleration of that enchondral growth. The classic examples are those of childhood *arthritis*, especially the disease known as juvenile rheumatoid arthritis in the USA and juvenile idiopathic arthritis internationally. Another example is the increased local maturation that results from the vascularity accompanying the absorbing of hemorrhage from *hemophilia* or

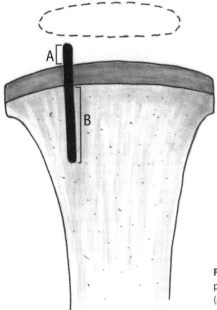

Fig. 37. Schematic of the ossified "hyphen" in the physis (*A*), which continues as a dense longitudinal line (*B*) in the metaphysis and into the shaft. A majority of children show at least one hyphen at radius or ulna.

other bleeding disorders. Because of the acceleration in maturation in hemophilia, epiphyses and their equivalents, including tarsals and carpals, not only overgrow, but also become irregular in pattern from the crowding of the overgrown centers (Fig. 38).

Interestingly, increased vascularity or growth in the knee region promotes medial greater than lateral growth in the proximal tibia epiphysis, causing relative valgus. For example, valgus may occur in a child beginning to rapidly resume growth after kidney transplantation.

Growth centers involved with much more than normal use because of specific athletic (or occupational) activity may overgrow compared to the normal or the contralateral size, presumably because of increased vascularity of the muscular activity.

The lack of any muscular activity in the region of a growing bone results in a lack of transverse growth (membranous bone), that is quite evident in polio, which is infantile paralysis of infectious etiology. Although the lower extremity bones are most often involved, the most recent case I have seen involved upper extremity polio resulting in a markedly narrow humerus. Similarly, lack of motion secondary to a childhood stroke may yield more slender bones on the affected side.

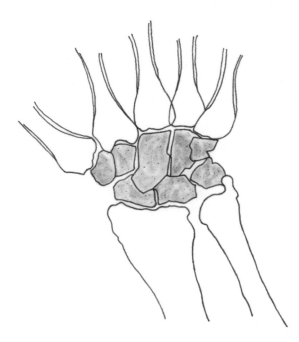

Fig. 38. Overgrowth and crowding of carpal bones at the wrist, typical for juvenile idiopathic arthritis (and for hemophilia as well). The longitudinal width of the carpus is decreased compared to normal despite the excessively rapid maturation. As the overgrown bones push against each other, the contours become irregular ("bizarro" shape), yet the surfaces become more congruent than normal with the neighboring bone, including the radio-carpal joints.

Because multiple (or solitary) cartilaginous exostosis in metaphyses results in a portion of that bone's enchondral physis being redirected to relatively transverse growth, the overall longitudinal growth of that bone is decreased. Therefore, with paired bones, the one with the more exostosis tends to be the shorter of the two (see Fig. 17).

Temporary or permanent epiphyseodesis, or hemipiphyseodesis, takes off enchondral growth of an entire or (hemi-) a portion of a growth plate. This allows the contralateral bone to catch up in length, or else allows straightening of an abnormal angle at an articulation.

Any tubular bone with multiple stippled epiphyses at its end tends to be shorter than expected in the shaft. This relative shortness, presumably from vascular supply decrease, persists when the epiphyseal stipples metamorphose into multiple epiphyseal dysplasia (the flatness of such involved epiphyses contribute somewhat to the overall shortness of the bone).

On the side of high vascularity from arthritis or fracture repair, growth arrest/recovery lines will be further from the physis from which they came, and which they parallel. Conversely, asymmetric closeness (or tethering) of those lines to the physis is a sign of decreased growth (from tethering or from low vascularity).

Melorheostosis in childhood consists of zones of increased bone density within bone, either shaft or growth center or both. Almost always, maturation of the involved bones is decreased and, in association, the bones and growth centers are decreased in size (Fig. 39). Adjacent joints may be clinically painful. (In adults, the condition known as melorheostosis has a different radiographic character, with candle-wax-like "dripping" of dense bone along the outside of shafts.)

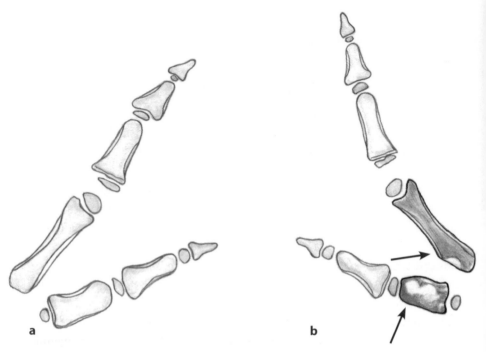

Fig. 39a,b. Melorheostosis (**b**) in childhood, compared to normal (**a**). Bones affected with the endosteal dense areas (arrows) tends almost always to be shorter than unaffected bones. The reason for decreased length likely relates to decreased vascularity.

11 Arthritis and Related Bone Disease

Abnormally increased vascularity means increased bone growth in childhood, especially enchondral growth. When long term hypervascularity affects a growth site or area, the result is an increase in maturation until such time as the growth plate [prematurely] fuses. The classic hypervascularity effect is the increased maturation related to arthritis, whether juvenile idiopathic arthritis [JIA] (which is still known as "JRA" in the USA), one of the enthesiopathies, or infectious arthritis. Especially in severe infectious arthritis, the possibility of destruction of a physis or acrophysis adds the possibility of the early elimination of a site of growth. Heat or electrical injury may also speed maturation only to be followed by early premature cessation of growth.

Most sites of JIA involve growth centers that are "encumbered," that is, they lie between other bony elements. As a result, the accelerated maturation results in crowding of the centers, giving them an abnormal, often angulated or squared-off shape. I speculate that the crowding leads to local decreased vascularity in the growth cartilage that is so squeezed (Fig 40). When the arthritis is unilateral at a level, comparison with the uninvolved side is helpful to show the advanced maturation as well as the altered contours (they resemble the angular contours of the "Bizarro" characters in Superman comics). When the hypervascularity is bilateral, comparison to bone age standard images may be helpful. Advanced bone age is another way of stating that centers are overgrown for age. Because of the crowding, articulating bones are typically more congruent than normal – or, otherwise stated, their contours fit more precisely the adjacent contours (Fig. 40).

Crowding does not affect unencumbered bones. Thus, the patella, except for its femoral margin, is unencumbered and can overgrow without crowding. The result is an enlarged "squared" appearing patella that is not shortened. Those margins of carpals most medial and most lateral (and most anterior and posterior) are not encumbered as are the other surfaces and should be less deformed by the crowding forces.

As maturation is accelerated, the growth cartilage surrounding ossification centers is being converted early to bone, so that the remaining cartilage is being used up; or, otherwise stated, the ossification center appears closer to the neighboring bones. For example, at the JIA-involved hip, the femoral growth center seems to be closer to the acetabular roof than normal; thus, the cartilage ("joint") space is narrower.

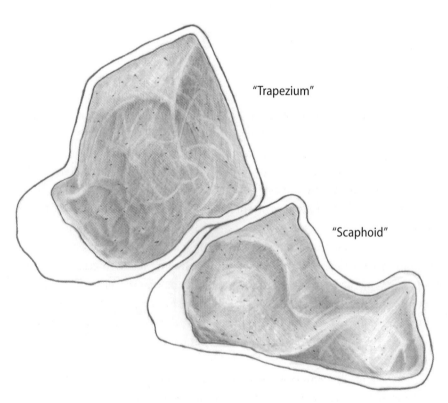

"Trapezium"

"Scaphoid"

Fig. 40. Juvenile idiopathic arthritis. As overgrown carpal bones get crowded from overgrowth, the growth cartilage of apposing surfaces tends to become squeezed and thus thinner, perhaps the explanation of the decrease in size of the carpus in the face of overgrowth of individual bones.

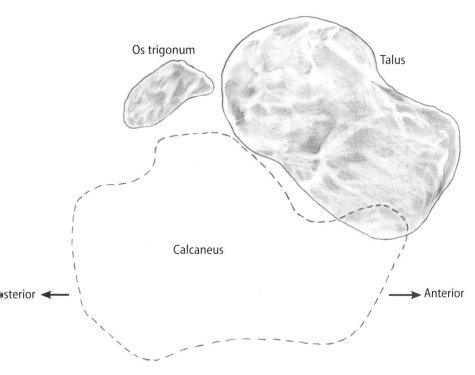

Fig. 41. In progressive pseudorheumatoid dysplasia, the unencumbered bony os trigonum center behind the talus ossifies earlier than normal and becomes considerably larger than normal (see Fig. 61 for normal os trigonum appearance)

In addition to arthritis, other causes of increased vascularity include the vascularity needed to remove blood from hemorrhage in hemophilia and other bleeding disorders. The advanced maturation and deformation of centers is quite similar in pattern to JIA. Healing of fractures entails increased vascularity; thus bones that have had fractures are often overgrown compared to the contralateral bone (unless the fragments are allowed to remain overlapped; however, the greater the fracture deformity, the more vascularity is needed for healing). Tumors may cause local hypervascular overgrowth. Enlarged growth centers are a feature of the higher vascularity of local athletic overuse of sites as well.

Pediatric growth centers are surrounded by considerable growth cartilage and thus are relatively protected from erosions due to JIA. Therefore, perceived irregularities of the margins on radiographs are more likely crowding-deformation than actual erosions.

The crowded wrist and other articular growth sites in Kniest disease and other megaepiphyseal skeletal dysplasias also have crowding and irregular shape of the involved centers

In *Albright syndrome,* which includes the bony and skin findings of fibrous dysplasia, bone maturation is accelerated. It seems as if the body is trying to end the problems ensuing from abnormal growth (including fractures) as soon as possible, by ending growth sooner than usual. Fractures through bone affected by fibrous dysplasia may become less frequent after maturity is achieved.

In *progressive pseudorheumatoid dysplasia,* the same pattern of overgrowth and crowding seen in juvenile idiopathic arthritis occurs from genetic causes rather than inflammatory disease. As a result, bone shape is altered in the absence of inflammation; certain aspects of enchondral growth seem accelerated and the child experiences the same effect of crowded overgrown centers that leads to abnormal shape of growth centers. Quite characteristic is the enlarged, early appearing, os trigonum center behind the talus (Fig. 41).

Increased vascularity means increased maturation. Conversely, decreased vascularity means decreased maturation. For example, the earliest radiographic finding in avascular necrosis of the hip (Legg Calvé Perthes) is a smaller than normal head of the femur (and bone age itself tends to be decreased in affected children). The decreased bone growth in polio is in part due to decreased muscular activity, but decreased vascularity may slow maturation as well. The smaller foot bones and growth centers in a club foot is associated with decreased arterial flow to those sites. In brachial plexus palsy, decreased muscular activity is associated with decreased maturation of growth centers not only at the humerus, but often at the elbow and wrist as well, again perhaps related to the decreased blood flow.

In the infant (and prenatal) condition of *multiple stippled epiphyses* (also known as chondrodysplasia punctata) stipples are seen within areas of growth cartilage. I believe these calcifications lie within that growth cartilage not yet committed into the shape of a growth plate and are due to avascular incidents leading to the calcification. The associated growth center (of epiphysis, apophysis, tarsal, or carpal) usually is quite delayed in maturation compared to non-affected centers. Tubular bones associated with epiphyses at their physeal (or nonphyseal) ends also tend to be short, whether rhizomelic, mesomelic, or acromelic. If the child survives long enough for the stipples to become incorporated into their ossified bones, the involved portion of epiphyses and their equivalents remain irregular and the pattern becomes one of ***multiple epiphyseal dysplasia***, while the shorted tubular bones remain short (Fig. 42). This paragraph could also have belonged in Chapter 8, Dysplasias and Dysostoses. However, the irregular bones of multiple epiphyseal dysplasia fit poorly with adjoining bones at their joints and may well cause early arthrosis.

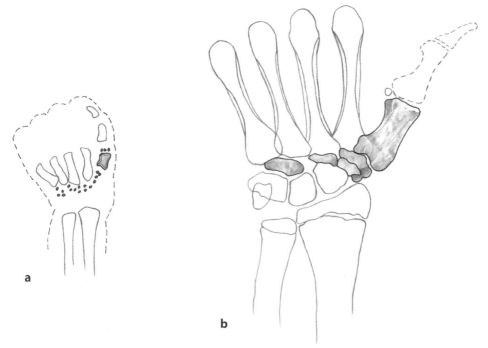

Fig. 42a,b. The natural consequence of multiple stippled epiphyses (**a**) is multiple epiphyseal dysplasia (**b**). Bones with the stipples (**a**) become deformed [here, the distal carpal row bones, for example] (**b**), and tubular bones with stipples [the 1st metacarpal in (**a**)] have shorter shafts both in infancy and later in development (**b**).

12

The "Ten Day Rule"

It takes ten days (well, maybe nine) *for periosteal reaction or bone destruction to appear on conventional radiographs.* This rule holds for infection, infarction, trauma, tumor, and other causes of callus or bone destruction. It holds for newborns as well as older children. The break in bone from fracture, of course, appears immediately (unless it is too subtle to be recognized). Thus, callus from a stress fracture, say of a tarsal bone, is seen only after nine days following the traumatic event that broke the camel's (trabeculum's) back.

- "Exception" No. 1: the lung side of ribs. An exception to the rule of ten days occurs following fracture (or infection, as well) of ribs: where the inner surface of a rib interfaces with the lung (Fig. 43), hematoma and then callus in formation is visible as a soft tissue-air interface long before ten days. However, no callus will be seen until ten days on the outer side of a rib interfacing with muscle and other soft tissue (Fig. 43).

- "Exception" No. 2: the zone of provisional calcification reappears well before ten days after successful treatment of nutritional rickets (see Fig. 20).

- "Exception" No. 3: in severe hyperparathyroidism, callus may not calcify sufficiently to be seen, even after ten days. I have knowingly encountered only one example.

Matrix vesicles are responsible for the appearance of bone-density calcification/ossification at ten days. Apparently, ten days and a proper calcium: phosphate ratio are necessary for matrix vesicles to sufficiently "do their thing." First empty matrix vesicles bud from the plasma membrane of chon-

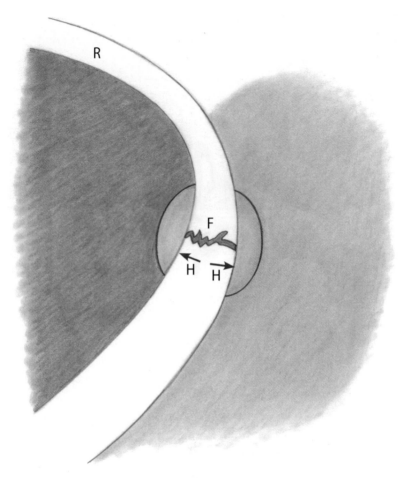

Fig. 43. Illustration of the rib-exception to the 10 day rule. The fracture (*F*) of rib *R* develops hemorrhage (*H*) beneath periosteum from the trauma. In soft tissue <u>outside</u> the rib (*light gray*), the hematoma is <u>not</u> seen on radiographs until it begins to calcify/ossify at about 10 days (soft tissue interfacing with soft tissue). However, within hours, the hematoma <u>is</u> visible on radiographs on the <u>inside</u> of the rib, being an interface between soft tissue and air of lung (shown here in *dark gray*).

drocytes, then they load calcium and phosphate ions, which then slowly align as calcium hydroxyapatite crystals. It takes a while to achieve all this, resulting in practice as the ten day rule before enough calcification is present to allow an observer to see on conventional radiographs.

Both enchondral (endosteal callus) and membranous (periosteal reaction) bone follow the ten day rule. The first evidence of stress fracture of tarsals (and sometimes metatarsals or even tibia or fibula if the images are not sufficiently perused) is usually endosteal callus after nine days; the tarsals have no periosteum so there can be no periosteal reaction.

Periosteal reaction can be detected earlier than ten days by modalities other than plain radiographs: bone scanning (after about a day), MRI, CT, and ultrasound for starters. Ultrasound doesn't easily reveal endosteal callus, but does show periosteal elevation once it occurs (Fig. 44).

On those rare occasions when periosteal reaction will join together two adjacent bones (ribs, for example), one can expect more than ten days to elapse before the union is visible on plain images. In bone lengthening procedures with distraction in which the periosteum is left in place between the osteotomized bone portions, one also expects to see bone filling the gaps after no fewer than ten days. In the dating of child abuse, presence of endosteal callus or periosteal reaction means that it has been ten days since the traumatic episode, except for Exception No. 1, listed above, i.e., soft tissue density on the lung side of ribs, which occurs much sooner. Also, one should not mistake physiologic periosteal reaction along the long bones, usually beginning between one- and six-months of age, for periosteal reaction from any abuse fracture of the same bone, lest the dating of the trauma be falsely considered ten days or more, when it is actually less.

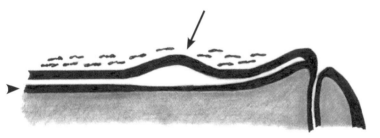

Fig. 44. The periosteal elevation (*arrow*) along the cortical shaft (*arrowhead*) of long bone can be easily seen on ultrasound imaging, even when not visible on radiographs (before subperiosteal reaction calcifies at about 10 days).

13 Paired Bones

The body has two featured sets of paired bones: the **radius and ulna** and the **tibia and fibula**. Other bones "in parallel" are the fingers and toes, the ribs, and even the vertebral column (and if you stretch the definition, the mandible and maxilla). This chapter discusses the principles of growth when one (or both) of a pair is disturbed. Some of these features apply as well to the other "in parallel" bones.

Most basically, if only one bone of a pair is shorter than usual, its mate is curved concave to the short bone (Fig. 45). It seems to be an attempt to maintain the location of the joints, although indeed the shorter bone may not reach one or both articulations with the next bone in line. Less commonly, a very short bone of a pair may not be associated with the bending of its mate. Chapter 14 discusses bowed bones in detail.

In multiple exostoses (osteochondromatosis), an exostosis of one of a bone pair may push upon the other bone, causing a concavity for the bump or other deformity (Fig. 46). Also, the bone with the larger exostosis or more numerous exostoses tends to be shorter than the other bone.

Congenital fusion of the proximal radius and ulna is typically associated with some bowing of the radius and almost obligatory radius dislocation (the axis of the proximal radius does not point to the middle of humerus capitulum). Other fusions of paired or in-parallel bones will have analogous effects on the growth of each bone. However, sometimes postfracture fusion of radius and ulna, and especially tibia and fibula, does not disturb overall growth of those bones, which lack of disturbance is more likely when a child becomes older.

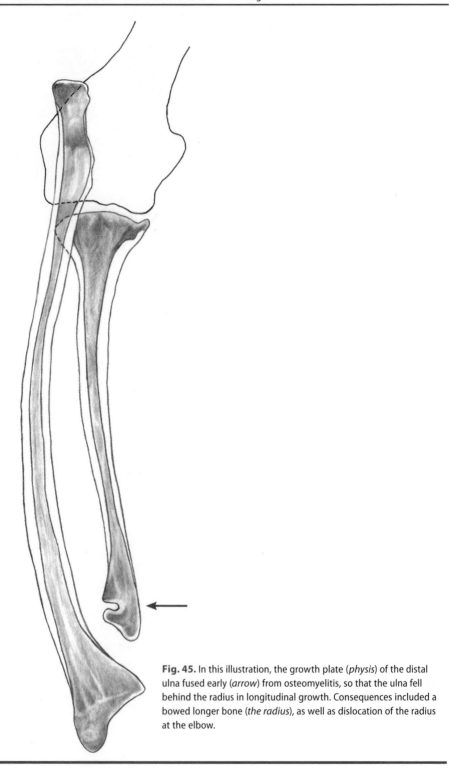

Fig. 45. In this illustration, the growth plate (*physis*) of the distal ulna fused early (*arrow*) from osteomyelitis, so that the ulna fell behind the radius in longitudinal growth. Consequences included a bowed longer bone (*the radius*), as well as dislocation of the radius at the elbow.

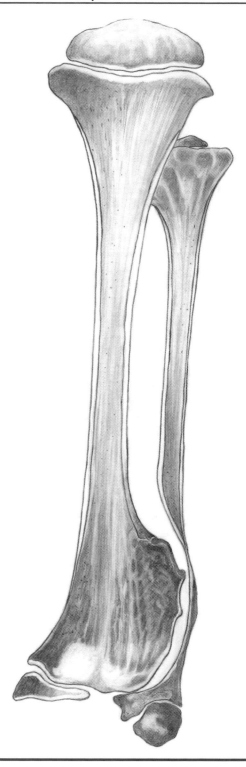

Fig. 46. In this subject with multiple exostoses, the large sessile exostosis of the distal tibia has, over time, pushed upon, narrowed, and deformed the adjacent fibula.

An interesting and sometimes clinically pertinent variation as to how hox genes guide the number and connectivity of ribs is the cervical rib/subjacent rib abnormality. In this situation (my guess would be that it is present in perhaps one out of 200 persons) one, or bilaterally both, of the uppermost ribs has a relatively vertical course that either closely approaches or actually fuses with a process coming up off the subjacent rib (Fig. 47). Other variations are a pseudarthrosis between them, or merely a local widening of the subjacent rib rather than a frank upward process. Once in a while, part of the brachial plexus or a vessel of the upper extremity is squeezed in the medial region bounded by the fused or nearly fused bones.

In vertical pedicle bar of the vertebral column, one or more pedicles is fused to the pedicle beneath it. If this happens only on one side, an unrelenting progressive scoliosis convex away from the side of the bar may be expected (Fig. 48), and early surgery is recommended. When the pedicles are so fused, no nerve root can exit between them and so the nerve rootlets are divided (presumably under the guidance of hox genes) among the next fora-

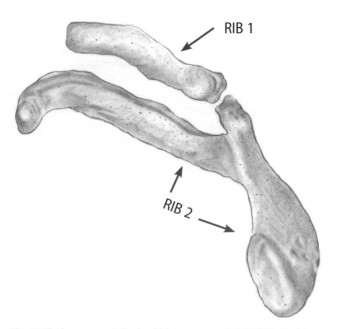

Fig. 47. The hox gene variation in which an uppermost rib "*RIB 1*" articulates or nearly fuses with an upward process from the subjacent rib "*RIB 2*". Some variation of this variation is present in about 1 of 200 individuals.

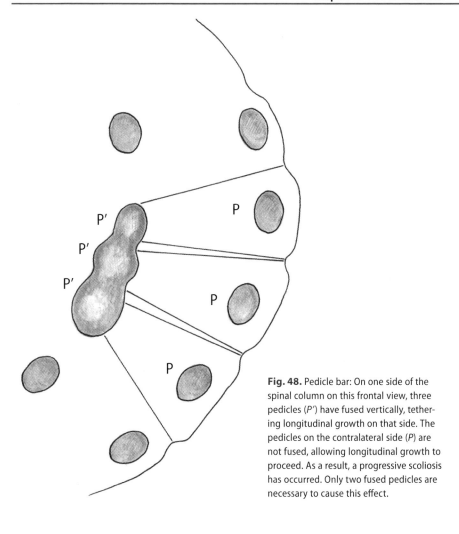

Fig. 48. Pedicle bar: On one side of the spinal column on this frontal view, three pedicles (*P'*) have fused vertically, tethering longitudinal growth on that side. The pedicles on the contralateral side (*P*) are not fused, allowing longitudinal growth to proceed. As a result, a progressive scoliosis has occurred. Only two fused pedicles are necessary to cause this effect.

men above and the next foramen below. Interestingly, scoliosis is not usually seen in the condition of congenital absence of a pedicle. In association with diastomatomyelia of the cord, often the lamina of the involved level is fused to a subjacent or suprajacent lamina.

In the situation of transverse carpal coalition fusion, such as lunate and triquetrum, which is generally a malformation of no consequence, one sees the actual bony fusion only later in development; earlier, the ossific centers appear increasingly closer together than normal as they mature.

In Apert syndrome, among some other polydactyly/syndactyly conditions, tubular bones may be fused proximally and separate again distally, or indeed fuse, separate, and then fuse again. Interestingly and unfortunately, premature fusion of cranial sutures occurs in Apert syndrome as well. For the patient, the ability to move fingers would seem more important than the resultant effects on longitudinal growth.

An unfortunate, curious hox gene variation of development is mirror image polydactyly in a hand or foot, in which a preaxial ray has all the other more postaxial rays on both sides of it, extending away from that ray in the middle (the example I have seen on clinical radiographs (Fig. 49) had a great toe in the middle of the foot, with a second toe on either side of it, and so on, until the two fifth toes appeared, giving nine toe rays in total. The foot and ankle had shorter and narrower bones than the normal contralateral foot. Before I read the technical explanation for the condition, I called it "toesis.")

If one of the mesomelic paired bones is miniscule or not formed at all, the other bone tends to be broad and may or may not be bowed.

Traumatic plastic bowing of the fibula may rarely prevent healing of a tibia shaft fracture. I have seen a case which required fibula osteotomy to allow the tibia fracture to heal many months after the injury.

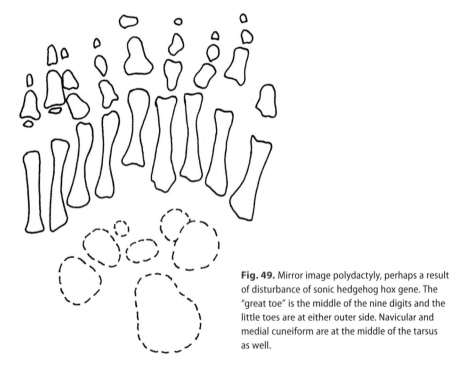

Fig. 49. Mirror image polydactyly, perhaps a result of disturbance of sonic hedgehog hox gene. The "great toe" is the middle of the nine digits and the little toes are at either outer side. Navicular and medial cuneiform are at the middle of the tarsus as well.

14

Bowed Bones

** this chapter actually covers two separate situations:

1. Bowing of Bones Themselves.
2. Bowing Secondary to Abnormal Fit of Articulating Bones at a Joint.

14.1 Bowing of Bones Themselves

Bowed bones have a convex/concave bend and thus are not as straight as normal.

Reasons for bone bowing include:

- *growth impairment in one of two paired bones*, leading to bowing of the shorter than normal bone;
  - a classic example is *Madelung deformity,* which is due to loss of medical growth at the distal radius physis, leading to ulna overgrowth as well as asymmetric radius growth, lateral greater than medial, and thus a bowed forearm (Fig. 50). The Madelung deformity may be congenital genetic as part of *dyschondrosteosis* or from acquired, usually traumatic damage to part of the distal radius physis. Otherwise, radius or ulna or tibia or fibula may have growth impaired from trauma or osteomyelitis, while its fellow bone is unaffected, leading to bowing of the longer (more normally growing) bone.

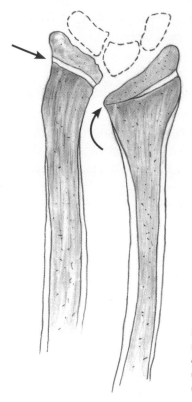

Fig. 50. Madelung deformity. The medial portion of the distal radius physis (*curved arrow*) is fused, tethering distal radius growth medially while growth continues laterally. Meanwhile, the unfused distal ulna physis (*arrow*) continues to grow, making the ulna longer than the radius.

- *walking with bones that are weakened*:
  - current or prior metabolic bone disease causing weakening, such as secondary hyperparathyroidism associated with rickets. Note that rickets changes at enchondral growing areas usually heal much sooner than the associated hyperparathyroidism;
  - healing of fractures while a limb is being used;
  - including fractures from osteogenesis imperfecta or from fibrous dysplasia (for example, the shepherd's crook lateral bow of the proximal femur shaft in fibrous dysplasia);
- angulation from fractures not in the plane of adjacent joint motion does not remodel as well as those in the plane;
- *traumatic plastic bowing.* A child's bones are more easily deformed than those of an adult. If a bone bends, but does not break, it may remain plastically deformed if the coefficient of plastic deformation is exceeded. Typically ulna, radius, or fibula is affected;

- Paget disease in the older adult, or its pediatric rare equivalent, *hyperphosphatasemia*, similarly may yield bowed bones from limb use.

- *intrauterine causes*:
  - prenatally and thereafter in *hypophosphatasia*, associated with skin dimple and perhaps Bowdler spurs extending to the dimple (see Fig. 15);
  - *camptomelic dysplasia* (also known, inappropriately, as campomelic dysplasia) receives its name from bowed bones in utero (mandible is small, cervical kyphosis present, small scapula and iliac bones, among other findings);
  - other in utero bowed bones, either genetic or from position/packing such as tibial kyphoscoliosis. Bending of tibia (and fibula, perhaps radius and ulna) in neurofibromatosis. Maternal hypoparathyroidism can lead to fetal hyperparathyroidism, which can lead to the bowing of long bones in utero, presumably from microfractures.

- *some genetic diseases with curved bones*:
  - the expanded (duplication of sorts) hamate in *Ellis van Creveld syndrome* protrudes medially distally (in the shape of a ham, thus the "ham-shaped hamate"; Fig. 51) and thus is curved;
  - in *Melnick Needles osteodysplasty*, ribs and tubular bones are ribbonlike or curved; even vertebral bodies may be somewhat misshapen;

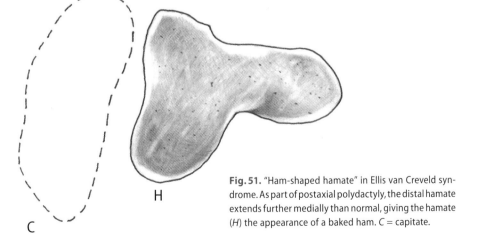

Fig. 51. "Ham-shaped hamate" in Ellis van Creveld syndrome. As part of postaxial polydactyly, the distal hamate extends further medially than normal, giving the hamate (*H*) the appearance of a baked ham. *C* = capitate.

- in *diastrophic dysplasia* the so-called hitchhiker thumb is short and often curved and the cervical spine is kyphotic, often markedly so (so don't forget a lateral image of the cervical spine when evaluating a child with this malformation syndrome);
- several *mesomelic dysplasias,* including Nievergelt, have curved tibias and often radiuses;
- ribs bending (from being longer than normal) in *Marfan* and other doliochostenomelias, resulting in pectus excavatum or carinatum

● *other:*
  - bowing from adjacent exostosis of a paired bone, or from asymmetric growth from the exostosis (or perhaps enchondroma) itself;
  - pectus excavatum and carinatum are curvings of sternum in sagittal plane;
  - *lateral clavicle hook,* a greater than normal concavity (smaller radius of curvature) downward at the lateral clavicle (Fig.52) when the arms are down against the chest (anatomic position); associated with reduction deformities of the ipsilateral upper extremity or with upper extremity weakness;
  - healing of valgus or varus osteotomy;
  - *foreshortening in space* by suboptimal positioning for x-ray (with the

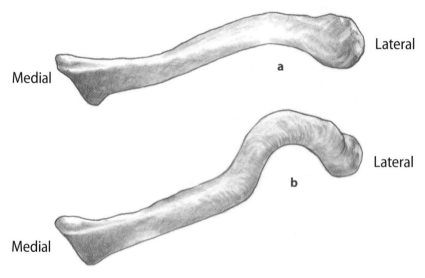

Fig. 52a,b. Compared to the normal (**a**), the lateral clavicle hook shows a greater than normal concavity (shorter radius of curvature) laterally (**b**). This pattern is associated with reduction deformities of the upper extremity bones or with muscular weakness of that extremity.

bone not parallel to the x-ray screen or plate) may exaggerate a normal metaphyseal curve (Fig. 53);
– frontal bossing as in achondroplasia is a forward bowing of the frontal bone.

– *VOLKMANN LAW: compression forces inhibit growth; tensile forces stimulate growth.* A bowed lower extremity bone, especially tibia, has a thicker cortex on the concave side in response to the forces of the Volkmann Law.

● 1′. *Bowing of teeth*
Abnormalities of growth or of life events of a tooth:
– pressure from adjacent bones or cysts or masses;
– **dilaceration** = curvature from trauma during development or occasionally idiopathic. Can be up to 90 degrees; most typically at the crown root junction. Orotrachial intubation has been implicated as a reason for trauma in premature infants, for example.

● 1″. *Bowing of finger or toe nails.* Since growth continues during adulthood, this is not limited to childhood.

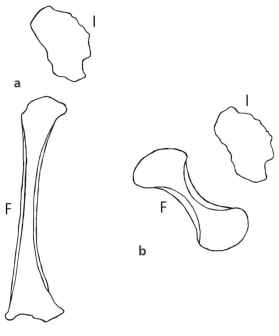

Fig. 53a,b. Foreshortening in space (**b**) compared to a normal femur appearance (**a**) in a kicking baby considerably flexing the hip. F = femur, I = iliac bone, frontal view. The shape of the foreshortened "in space" bone resembles the shortened bone of metatropic dysplasia (see Fig. 31), which is foreshortening "in time" from slowed enchondral growth.

14.2 Bowing Secondary to Abnormal Fit of Articulating Bones at a Joint

Bowing is also used to describe an extremity part that is bent at one or more joints secondary to the abnormal shape of the articulating bones at a joint (thus, clinodactyly, a medial convexity of the little finger, is associated with a short middle phalanx with a trapezoidal shape, longer medially than laterally. [Quiz question: Is this a varus or a valgus deformity];

- genu varum of the knees, so nicely termed "O legs" in German. Genu valgum, or "X legs" in German (Fig. 54);
- scoliosis
  - idiopathic, for which theories abound;
  - asymmetric muscle pull (classically, after neuroblastoma unbalanced radiation);
  - congenital, associated with lateral hemivertebra or other segmentation abnormalities of the vertebral column;
  - torticollis, most often in infancy due to sternocleidomastoid muscle thickening giving positional abnormality; otherwise consider segmentation anomaly of the vertebral column.
- kyphosis
  - congenital associated with posterior hemivertebra;
  - cervical in camptometic dysplasia, diastrophic dysplasia, some Larsen syndrome, and following laminectomy in neurofibromatosis-1;
  - Scheuermann adolescent kyphosis.
- hallux valgus and its equivalent varus deformity of the fifth ray, the bunionette.
- The **delta phalanx**, or **longitudinally bracketed diaphysis**, is an abnormality of a short tubular bone in which the epiphysis curves around along the shaft (diaphysis) and thus creates some enchondral bone growing transversely instead of longitudinally (Fig. 55). Such bones are generally short. In the "kissing delta phalanges" anomaly, the bone is duplicated, with the longitudinal growth plate portions facing each other in mirror image fashion. Among other conditions with delta phalanges, consider Rubinstein Taybi syndrome.
- elbow, ankle, etc, varus/valgus after partial growth arrest from trauma;
- segmentation anomalies of finger, toes, mesomelic bones;

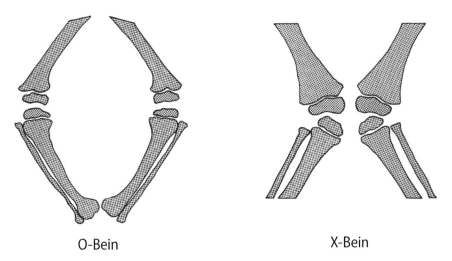

O-Bein   X-Bein

Fig. 54. The German term for knock knees (knee valgus) is the appropriate "X" legs; for bowlegs (knee varus) it is the appropriate "O" legs. From Oestreich AE: How to Measure Angles from Foot Radiographs, a Primer. Reprinted 1999 MLC, Cincinnati, p 9.

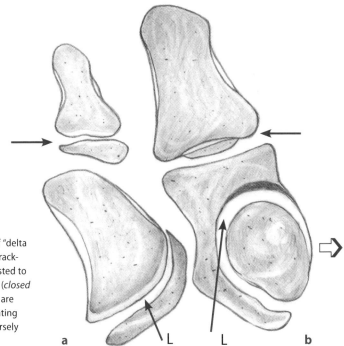

Fig. 55a,b. Two examples of "delta phalanx" or "longitudinally bracketed diaphysis (L)." As contrasted to customary transverse physes (*closed arrows*), these growth plates are abnormally longitudinal, creating uncustomary growth transversely (*open arrow*).

- asymmetric growth in frostbite, Kashin Beck, ratbite, see Chapter 10;
- bony bar (including vertical pedicle bar; see Fig. 48), staples across one side of a physis, radiation damage to part of a physis, increased asymmetric tibia growth from healing fracture or emerging from renal-caused growth retardation.

15 Alignment Abnormality

Alignment or positional relationships of the lower extremity are to be evaluated only from weight-bearing views.

For the definition of varus and valgus, Figure 56 from our little book, *How to Measure Angles from Foot Radiographs*, can be helpful. The terms refer to the relationship of a distal part of a limb with respect to a proximal part. The proximal part is considered as if it were in anatomic position, with the distal part's angular relation to that proximal part constant, despite the (mental) repositioning of the proximal part to that anatomic position. When we used films, that repositioning was done merely by turning the film. Now, then, when the distal part is directed more medial than normal in this positional set-up, the relationship is *varus*, whereas if it is directed as being more lateral than normal, it would be *valgus*. The result for the right hip yields the mnemonic (Fig. 57) reproduced here from our prior books, including *How to Measure Angles from Foot Radiographs*.

In *equinus* (horse-like position), the relationship (in weight-bearing or simulated weight-bearing) of the calcaneus to the tibia is disturbed, with the front of the calcaneus relatively tipped downward (Fig. 58). What semantic confusion: when the front of a calcaneus has the opposite of equinus in its relationship to the tibia, it is called a *calcaneus* deformity, and thus, a calcaneus calcaneus. Flat foot, or *pes planus*, is a low arch in weight-bearing. A *cavus* foot is a high arch, and a *rockerbottom* foot is a reversed, downwardly convex arch.

If one peripheral part of a growth plate is impaired in its growth, then an angulation develops as the remainder of the physis (or acrophysis) allows normal growth. Similarly, if the central portion of a physis is impaired, the

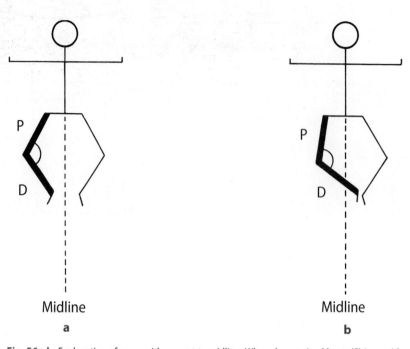

Fig. 56a,b. Explanation of varus with respect to midline. When the proximal bone (*P*) is considered as if in anatomic position (**b**), then the distal bone (*D*) heads more toward (across) the midline than normal, which is varus. From Oestreich AE: How to Measure Angles from Foot Radiographs, a Primer. Reprinted 1999 MLC, Cincinnati, p 2.

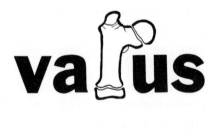

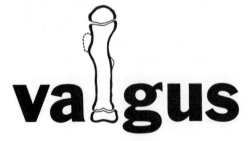

Fig. 57. Artist's mnemonic for varus and valgus of the right hip , from Oestreich AE: Pediatric Radiology, Medical Outline Series, 3rd ed., 1984 Medical Examination, New Hyde Park, NY, p 192.

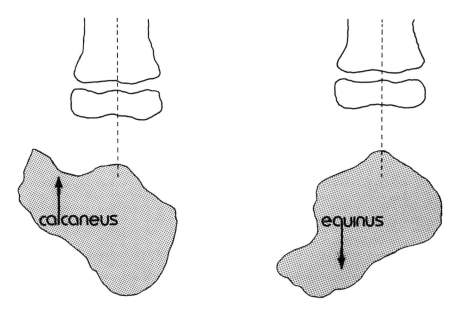

Fig. 58. Artist's mnemonic for equinus and calcaneus position of the calcaneus (os calcis). Weight-bearing images. In equinus, the anterior end of the bone tilts downward on lateral image, like the "q" of equinus dips down below the other consonants at the front of the word. In calcaneus, the anterior end of the bone lifts more upward than normal, like the "l" of calcaneus extends upward above the other consonants at the front of the word. From Oestreich AE, Crawford AH: Atlas of Pediatric Orthopedic Radiology. 1985, Georg Thieme, Stuttgart, p 115.

result is a coned-shaped epiphysis, in which the non-growing portion of the epiphysis seems to sink in to the metaphysis (actually, it is fixed while the more peripheral portions continue to grow).

Asymmetric neuromuscular activity may lead to asymmetric bone growth. A classic example of asymmetric muscle pull is the hip in neuromuscular weakness, affecting the abductors and adductors differentially, resulting in valgus femur and often subluxation of the hip as well.

Bowlegs is physiologic up to about 18 months of age (give or take a few months). When the abnormal compressive forces on the medial proximal tibia physis from ambulating on bow legs becomes too severe, ***Blount disease***, tibia vara of the young, may occur, slowing the medial physeal growth while lateral growth proceeds apace (Fig. 59). As a result, bowing increases, setting up a vicious circle in which the deformity tends to increase as a result of the angulation. Surgical correction may be needed. Some degree of genu valgum, or **knock knees**, is physiologic for many years beginning at about 18 months of age.

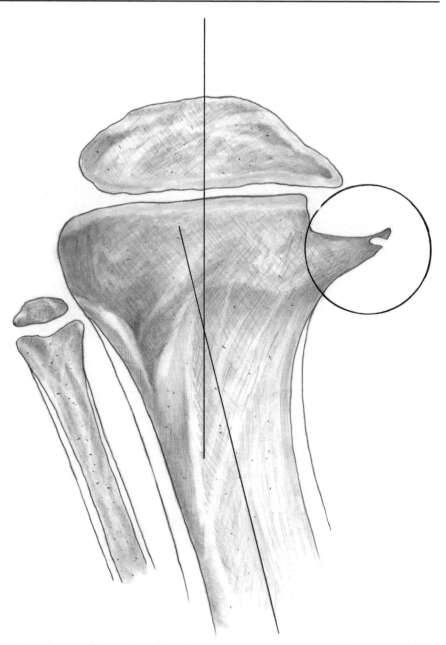

Fig. 59. Tibia vara of Blount disease. Related to impaired enchondral growth medially at the knee (*circled area*), a varus relationship (see *straight lines*) develops between the longitudinal axes of the tibia epiphysis and the tibia shaft (as well as fibula shaft).

16 Specific Characteristics of Specific Bones

I have always wanted to write something about the *vomer*, so here is my chance.

Except for persons involved with cleft palate and its repair, along with astute neuroradiologists, very few people know much about the vomer beyond its name and perhaps its location. The vomer is a flat bone which grows by membranous ossification. I assume that, like the skull flat bones at their sutures, the vomer grows at its outer margins by membranous ossification, as well (Fig.60).

The *coccyx* is another "neglected" bone about which it would be nice to say at least something. Unlike much of the sacrum, no lateral bone (such as the ilium for the sacrum) interacts with it or protects it. Children who bump that area of the body from abrupt termination of progress down a snowy or icy decline may injure that unprotected bone or its articulation with the sacrum. An acute sacrococcygeal kyphosis may be traumatic in origin; however, how did it look before the trauma? Unlike many of our fellow mammals, the human coccyx does not extend into a tail. However, a bulge or fold at the coccygeal level is sometimes seen in metatrophic dysplasia, analogous to a tail to those with an imagination.

The *middle phalanx of little finger* is often short; sometimes with a cone epiphysis and is frequently associated with clinodactyly (medial convexity), especially if the phalanx is trapezoidal in shape. Shortness is rarely associated with longitudinally bracketed diaphyses in the delta phalanx anomaly. Persons with a short middle phalanx of the little finger tend to have a somewhat lower adult height than those having the normal length of that bone, an interesting statistical correlation.

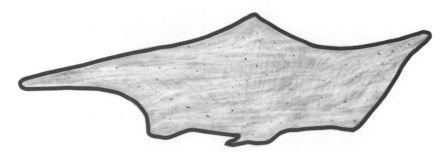

Fig. 60. a vomer, side view. All growth at margins (*blue*) and on surfaces is membranous.

The *os trigonum* center behind the talus has a curious history during child-hood, which we have investigated. By the way, around here we pronounce the name of this center as if it were "Oestreich-onum," with Oestreich pro-nounced "Oh Strike." Virtually all children who have a normal talus develop an os trigonum center behind the talus in the latter portion of the first decade of life (Fig. 61a), girls about a year earlier than boys, and that center fuses to/into the posterior talus within about a year (Fig. 61b). Let us call that enchon-dral center the os trigonum 1. Then in the early part of the second decade of life, or sometimes a bit later, a second os trigonum center, the os trigonum 2 (Fig. 61c), appears in a much smaller percentage of children, perhaps between 10% and 20%; it sometimes eventually fuses, but not always. Occasionally the os trigonum 1 or 2 may ossify from more than one center. The os trigonum acts somewhat like an apophysis (analogous to the posterior apophysis of the calcaneus) since it is not between bones; however, it is not tugged upon by any tendon.

The *distal phalanx of the great toe and the thumb* is broad in the Rubin-stein Taybi Syndrome and in the Robinow syndrome. In each case, it acts as a forme fruste of duplication. This broad distal phalanx of both great toe and thumb may have a distal "notch" (a minor form of apoptosis) or a distal midline "hole" in Rubinstein Taybi (Fig. 62) and may well have side by side duplicated distal portions in Robinow. In Rubinstein Taybi, the distal tufts of fingers and toes 2 through 5, tend to be broader than normal.

In *myositis ossificans progressiva*, abnormalities of the great toes are always seen and may be the key to the diagnosis before the myositis or fibro-sitis ossifies. The first metatarsal and its proximal phalanx are malformed or even fused. The first metacarpals also tend to be short.

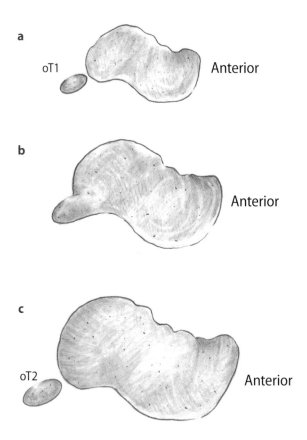

Fig. 61a–c. The 2 os trigonum centers behind the talus. In the later first decade of life, almost universally an os trigonum (*oT1*) appears (**a**); then fuses with the talus in about a year (**b**). Then in the second decade of life, 10–20% of individuals develop a second os trigonum center (*oT2*) (**c**), which may or may not eventually fuse to the talus.

The *lateral clavicle hook* was first described by Igual [Igual M, Giedion A.: The lateral clavicle hook: its objective measurement and its diagnostic value in Holt Oram syndrome, diastrophic dwarfism, thrombocytopenia-absent radius syndrome and trisomy 8. Ann Radiol (Paris). 1979, 22:136-41]. It is a greater than normal upward convexity of the lateral clavicle when the subject's arms are at the side. It is seen when a reduction deformity occurs in the ipsilateral upper extremity or in the presence of muscular weakness, including brachial plexus palsy (see Fig. 52).

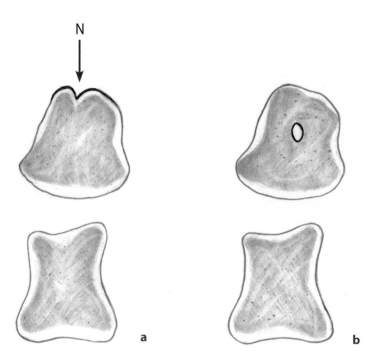

Fig. 62a,b. Schematic of two versions of great toe (or thumb) distal phalanges in Rubinstein Taybi syndrome (RTS). In each, the distal phalanx is short and broad. The proximal phalanx may be short as well. In many RTS subjects (**a**), a notch (*N*) appears between two hemi-heads of the wide phalanx. In other RTS subjects (**b**), a hole is seen between the two hemi-necks of the broad distal phalanx.

Subject Index